# YOGA
# *beyond Fitness*

# YOGA beyond Fitness

*Getting More than Exercise from an Ancient Spiritual Practice*

TOM PILARZYK, PH.D.

QUEST

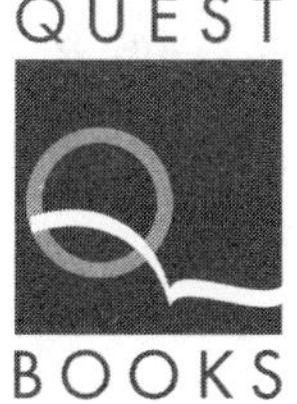

BOOKS

Theosophical Publishing House
Wheaton, Illinois • Chennai, India

First Quest edition 2008



Quest Books
Theosophical Publishing House
P.O. Box 270
Wheaton, IL 60187-0270

www.questbooks.net

Cover image: © Duncan Smith/Corbis
Cover design, book design, and typesetting by Dan Doolin

Chapter six elaborates upon ideas first appearing in the April 2005 issue of *Sacred Pathways Magazine* as "Yoga at a Crossroads." Chapter fourteen appears in earlier form as "The Quiet Rebellion" in the August 2005 issue of *Synchronicity Magazine*. Chapter seventeen is an extended version of an article in *YogaChicago Magazine*, February 2005. Chapter twenty appears in a shortened version in *YogaChicago Magazine*, August 2005. Chapter twenty-two appears in slightly abbreviated form in the April 2006 issue of *Yogi Times*.

Library of Congress Cataloging-in-Publication Data

Pilarzyk, Thomas, Ph.D., RYT.
Yoga beyond fitness: getting more than exercise from an ancient spiritual practice / Thomas Pilarzyk.—1st Quest ed.
p. cm.
Includes bibliographical references and index.
ISBN 978-0-8356-0863-3
1. Yoga. 2. Spiritual life. 3. Title.
B132.Y6P495 2008
204'.36—dc22 2008013957

Printed in the United States of America

5 4 3 2 1 * 08 09 10 11 12

*To those who live Yoga and*
*honor its transformative nature*

# CONTENTS

*Part 3*

## TRANSFORMING SELF

# PREFACE

I began writing this book after returning from a yoga training session in New England. Seated on my couch the morning after, I recalled the story of a fellow practitioner who had been assaulted many years before and had learned to forgive and even love her aggressor. Her story embodied for me the raw healing power that Yoga manifests through a widened heart. With time, telling stories of how Yoga transforms us sprouted from that memory. Emboldened by love, open to vulnerability, and informed by a pinch of insight, I began to transfer experience onto paper. My writing would continue over the next three years as I reflected on my roles as teacher, student, and observer of this path.

Although I loved Yoga, I realized in shaping my chapters that I felt some ambivalence toward it. Yoga is my transformative helm, anchor, map, and compass. Yet it has expanded over the decades to become a full-fledged industry of the contemporary marketplace, filled with so many producers, sellers, and consumers that they seem to outnumber the spiritual teachers, healers, and devoted adepts. This phenomenon, I surmised, exposes an interesting bipolar condition—where twenty-five-year-old flexiphiles attracted to the newest yoga style and silver-haired masters of depth and breadth are creating a distinctively North American offspring of a sacred dance. Certainly, this represented a subject worthy of study.

Delving deeper, I also recognized how much I appreciate the business side of yoga. It allows me to read insightful books and magazines on topics I love, to travel to mountain retreat centers for practice opportunities, to meet gifted teachers from whom I learn so much, and to buy products where a portion of profit is donated to global causes. It is the balance—or more properly, the tangible imbalance—that began to concern me most as principle, priority, and pathway seemed to erode little by little with each passing day. Was yoga merely a fitness industry masquerading as spirituality, as Yoga?

Book authors and magazine editors, retreat directors and studio owners, and physicians and yoga therapists now seem to be grappling with finding a middle ground for modern American yoga. This middle ground lies somewhere between a growth-is-good mentality—that more Americans have an opportunity to practice and improve their health, fitness, and well-being—and a recognizable unease that Yoga's deeper transformative experiences are being drowned out by its reduction to "doing the poses" among a growing customer base. Any authentic spiritual path would appear to be in crisis whenever giving consumers what they want supersedes its ability to maintain the deeper metaphysical message for serious practitioners.

Practicing Yoga is challenging, but not in the way that the more superficial side of the discipline indicates. When we think of yoga, most of us may think first of the difficulty of particular poses or of remaining committed to certain practice routines. Yet it is how we are guided by the Yogic roadmap off the mat that counts most—reconnecting with a daily intention; checking our seated posture; watching the turning of our minds and the straying of our thoughts; welcoming difficult situations that test our resolve to stay present; remaining openhearted when it is too easy to close down emotionally; reminding ourselves to breathe deeply, stay with the flow of energy, and witness the spontaneous play of activity around us; and respecting teachings that are both plausible and possible to attain. These actions are Yoga's touchstones, helping us live more fully, happily, healthily, and in concert with the energy of the world. Yet they can be compromised at a moment's notice.

What a challenge *this* Yoga can be! I often find myself stumbling along the path I try to follow. So I metaphorically pick myself back up again and again and start all over. The last conclusion that I would ever draw from my decades-long exercise is that it is meant to be easy. But it *does* get easier with time as I learn to live with more spontaneity and surrender and even with a bit more grace. Doing the poses is my personal training ground for this deeper application of Yoga to my life.

So this is not a "how to" book where yoga is the object of technical inquiry—how to do the poses and breath work to feel or look better. Nor is it a spiritual discourse on Yoga or an analysis of the path's philosophical tenets. Many wonderful works by T. K. V. Desikachar, Georg Feuerstein, B. K. S. Iyengar, Srivatsa Ramaswami, Satchidananda, and others already fulfill those needs.[1] Rather, this book provides evidence that integrating Yoga into one's life is both a challenge and a blessing, much as Donna Farhi's *Bringing Yoga to Life*, Stephen Cope's *The Wisdom of Yoga*, and Elizabeth Gilbert's *Eat, Pray, Love* all do.

However, *Yoga beyond Fitness* also makes one unique contribution. It introduces the world of contemporary American yoga to those just discovering it or to those having practiced for a while who feel that something is amiss and that there is a deeper meaning that is readily accessible but not directly evident. In this sense, the book is both a sober wake-up call about how Yoga is being transformed and a hopeful, heartfelt tribute to its highest aspirations. As Yoga changes, its story is told through the experiences of those who practice and have been transformed by it. This book looks at Yoga as a phenomenon that deserves warm appreciation but also pause for reflection.

## Caught in the Middle

Yoga in North America was originally a coastal and mountain discipline, with more centers in large cities than in the rural countryside. While there are plenty of yoga studios today in Missouri, Indiana, and Minnesota, they are still overshadowed by the sheer range of opportunities for practice in places like California, New York, and Colorado. As a student of Yoga and meditation with over a twenty-year commitment to each, I have lived my entire life in some part of America's Great Midwest and have traveled to quench my thirst for these practices. As a result, sometimes I feel as if I must have a case of "Midwestern malaise," an ill-ease resulting from the fact that the Midwest is slightly off-center on the national yoga map.

Here is a case in point: A few years ago, a book profiling many of America's prominent Yoga and meditation teachers included just one current Midwesterner, from Cincinnati. The teachers were almost exclusively from the Northeast and West, despite the fact that a recent survey estimates that half of all yoga practitioners live elsewhere, within America's inner expanse.[2]

Regardless of where we live, our inner and outer worlds subtly reflect each other. I enjoy traversing the outer world to explore my inner one more deeply, whether I do Taos yoga or Alpine meditation. I know that I am not unique and that there are many of us for whom internal and external travel are one and the same trip, if we realize it or not. However, this book, a personal and sociological journey through the yoga scene today, is written from my slightly skewed Midwestern vantage point. Being a Midwesterner supposedly means that "what you see is what you get" without much pretension. There may be something to this down-to-earthiness and our attempt to hold to a more stable middle ground.

Perhaps my Midwestern perspective provides some healthy distance from the hot spots of cultural trendsetting to allow me to focus more on what is essential and what endures. Distance, after all, can offer a healthy perspective from which to explore thoughts and feelings about relationships. This book, driven by my love for practice, explores America's relationship—its modern love affair—with yoga. It is personal, because it draws upon the intimate experiences of teachers and students of this ancient path, including my own. It is sociological, since it stands back to explore the wider forces and interpersonal contexts shaping yoga as a phenomenon today and yielding consequences that cannot be clearly foreseen. These two strands—personal and social—are interwoven throughout the book, between the big and small picture of American yoga life, to create a tapestry that is at once particular and universal. In this way, yoga is both *my* story and *our* story.

## My Story of Yoga

My cross-fertilizing involvement with both Hinduism and Buddhism informs this book. My intellectual interest began with Hinduism, as did my dedication to Yoga. My commitment to meditation began with Buddhism. These two great practice traditions of Indian origin are dedicated to overcoming suffering through specific techniques of mind, body, and heart that promise to emancipate the practitioner through direct perception and experimentation. While their teachings are complementary, their explanations can vary. This book does not address their differences as much as it celebrates similarities. Any misunderstanding or misrepresentation is a product of my blurred vision and not of their legacies to transcendental understanding.

My perspective reflects a marriage of experiences with both as well as familiarity with Western social science. Decades ago, I was a graduate student interested in "alternative religions" who put down roots in the Upper Midwest and elsewhere in the country. I studied Hare Krishnas in Evanston and Divine Light Mission devotees in Chicago, spent time with Himalayan Institute members in Milwaukee and Transcendental Meditation practitioners in Madison, and sought out a range of others, here and there. I witnessed how the fervor and commitment of their college-aged converts transformed lives through practices that cultivate a love and knowledge for living fully and happily. Yes, there was plenty of confusion, unquestioned deference to authority, and the occasional instance of exploitation. But these young men and women grew up to become part of the wider culture; some are now the leaders of a broad movement in transformative consciousness that has influenced part of the cultural mainstream.

Eventually, I committed myself to meditation inspired by the teachings of Tibetan Buddhism. My daily and personal yoga ran parallel to my meditation. Years after first studying Hinduism, yoga would evolve into my life practice—the poses and breath work, ethical restraints and observances, dietary restrictions and chants, and meditation and visualization practices. So while this book has its origins in the interests of a young academic, it reaches fuller flower only in the later writings of a middle-aged adult who tries to apply its practices and teachings to his daily life. It is both as participant and observer that Yoga has become an important part of my personal story.

## Yoga's American Story

However, this book is much more than my own story. Yoga is all around us, and it is undergoing rapid change today. Classes seem to be everywhere, filled with yogas of the superficial and the profound. There are few maps to guide us in this buyer's marketplace, where it is not initially apparent if the producers and sellers themselves realize what they are doing to the product. While there are more opportunities for us to find a practice that fits our interests and needs, yoga has become a major commercial and medical venture. The resulting confusion over Yoga's underlying message seems to blow like the fog rolling off one of North America's Great Lakes, obscuring our vision for a time. The meaning of Yoga has less to do with holding *virabhadrasana 2* for a few minutes or with bringing your chest to the floor in *upavista konasana*, and much more to do with applying its broad, deep teachings to one's life—as that overly used phrase suggests—both on and off the mat.

# Preface

*Yoga beyond Fitness* attempts to capture the story of American yoga practice today, with special attention given to those who treat it with reverence or who wish to explore it as a receptacle of transformative power. What is happening to *our* Yoga as it becomes a pop culture discipline? What challenges await national yoga magazines, mountain retreat centers, and neighborhood studios trying to turn a healthy profit while remaining true to Yoga's underlying promise? What changes are coming to *kirtan*, the powerful, prayerful chanting informed by Yoga, in an entertainment-driven world? What does this all mean for our own experiences in class? To explore these and other questions, this book captures life away from the polished floorboards, rubberized mats, and props. It is about being challenged to transform our lives when victimized, when worn down or surprised by love and relationship, and when traveling in unfamiliar territory. It involves meeting a loved one at their death as a yogi. And more.

Since *Yoga beyond Fitness* relies on the stories of real human beings, their integrity and privacy deserve protection. I relied on taped interviews and shared quotes and context to ensure accuracy, or I drew on previously published interviews in which individuals are quoted (citations are provided in the notes section). In both cases, I used real names and am grateful for their contributions to my book. In a few situations, I created composite characters with fictitious names while sticking closely to the truth of actual experiences. Where Sanskrit terms appear, they are associated with corresponding English concepts, and their spelling is Anglicized (e.g., *āsana* becomes *asana*). When referring solely to a holistic spiritual path, as I do in the second and third sections of the book, the term "Yoga" is capitalized. Where it represents varied motivations for practice or one among many forms, as it does in the first section, yoga appears in lowercase.

Like our lives, this book ebbs and flows as shared and personal, universal and concrete. My hope is that one of these stories sweeps the reader like they have taken me, just as those windstorms blowing off the Great Plains reenergize and refertilize our land. After all, that is what Yoga is about—an incremental, transformative movement from our center, riding the storm within and without, experiencing energy and awareness flowing from our heart, one place from which our lives touch each other to make a difference.

*Yoga beyond Fitness* is dedicated to those who have a healthy yoga practice but do not live "near the action"—whether it be in the middle of Kansas, the desert country of Nevada, or the woodlands of Wisconsin. While we may travel to California's Spirit Rock Meditation Center or Massachusetts's Kripalu Center, our inner landscapes are not really different from one another or from the outer terrain. Like our minds, these landscapes remain deficient only if we perceive and affirm them to be so, and if those with some influence do likewise. These inner and outer terrains quite literally remain the fertile ground for practice. We gain release from any malaise once we realize that, fundamentally, here *is* where the action is, after all—in any and every circumstance in which we find ourselves. To come to this realization is to step beyond what is superficial into a deeper, more vibrant world where Yoga becomes a path, a life practice.

# ACKNOWLEDGMENTS

I am indebted to those who encouraged me, knowing that this book remained close to my heart. I am convinced that, without Julie Wichman's guidance and Beverly Pilarzyk's support, these words would not appear in print. I am also thankful to those who provided wise counsel and thoughtful reviews. Dean Lesser, Ph.D., and Michael Carroll, CYT, offered invaluable feedback on an early draft. Jane McAdams' careful reading of a later draft helped to clarify my words and refine their meaning. Others furnished insightful suggestions on selected portions, including Lakshmi Bharadwaj, Ph.D., Kelly McGonigal, Ph.D., David Shapiro, M.D., Anthony Kubicki, M.S., and Roxanne Johnson, J.D.

I also wish to acknowledge those who gave of their time and energy to be interviewed for the various chapters. They are the voices who make Yoga come alive and will assure that it remains a path of joy and light, healing and compassion, in a darkened and increasingly troubled world. While grateful to all contributors, the opinions and conclusions expressed in this book remain my own.

INTRODUCTION

# APPROACHING THE MAT

It seems everyone is doing yoga. The yoga explosion hit the country by 2000, and Americans have been practicing in growing numbers ever since. You can now go virtually anywhere in a metropolitan area and find a class. Yoga is even offered by businesses, not to mention in private homes. Universities are teaching classes, too, along with fitness and recreation centers, churches, and schools. Classes are regularly advertised in local papers, newsletters, fliers, and posters. City yoga magazines have entered the market, and teacher-training programs number well over four hundred on the national registry of the Yoga Alliance, an umbrella organization setting standards and promoting certified instructors.

An estimated sixteen million people currently practice and spend roughly six billion dollars annually on classes, products, and services, according to a 2008 Harris Interactive poll.[1] Mediamark Research found that three million in 2006 practiced at least twice a week.[2] Yoga's visibility exposes its diversity and the varied reasons people are turning to it. Although it originated on the Indian subcontinent some five thousand years ago as a path of spiritual liberation, today yoga has become a tool for feeling fit and looking good, dealing with stress, and recovering from ill-health, injury, or surgery.

Yoga's burst in popularity results partly from national and local trends. Continuous media emphasis on youth, health, and beauty, as well as the many celebrities and health professionals touting yoga's physical benefits, certainly have played a role in leading us to gyms, fitness centers, and studios, as have our stressful, fast-paced lives of nanoseconds and sound bites. Meanwhile, the growth in expendable incomes fed by an expanding economy at the turn of the past century also made its contribution. According to the U.S. Census, many cities witnessed a positive inflow of young professionals—key yoga consumers. The result is that "yoga" yields over ninety-three million entries on a Google search, Target sells yoga mats, and a monthly pass at one New York City studio exceeds three hundred dollars.

On a deeper level, yoga's popularity is fed by its own inner dynamic, ever-challenging techniques and expanding styles that naturally open and unify body, mind, and heart. Pandit Rajmani Tigunait, head of the Himalayan International Institute of Yoga Science and Philosophy, explains yoga's intrinsic effects this way: "It unblocks energy which then starts flowing everywhere throughout the body. All your limbs and organs, including your nervous system, brain, and mind are nourished, so you feel good."[3] Different forms of yoga have the potential to bring about this change as we draw attention to the breath, synchronized with our movement.

Yoga is best known for increasing flexibility through those pretzel-like poses or postures known as "*asanas.*" At first blush, their ancient Sanskrit names appear exotic: *mandalasana, sirsasana*, and *trikonasana*. They take their meanings from nature, human creativity, and archetypal roles—mountain, tree, fish, crow, bridge, dancer, hero, and warrior. With time, students learn the symbols, if not the pronunciations. But yoga also strengthens and lengthens, promoting endurance while working with breath and awareness through *pranayama*—techniques for engaging life-force energy, or *prana*, which, according to yogis, rides on our breath. Poses and breath work are major elements of *Hatha*, what most Americans today associate with the term "yoga."

Yoga's effect can mirror that of conventional physical workouts. Confronting a daily sensory overload, multitasking at work, and feeling a need to balance our busy lives, many of us experience stress, anxiety, or depression. We may live so fully in our overactive minds that we feel disengaged from our bodies, with less-than-healthy eating habits and critical self-judgments to boot. In reaction, some of us may adopt machine-like workouts that repetitiously whip and pound our bodies into shape that do, in fact, achieve positive outcomes—like keeping our cardiovascular systems in optimal condition, shedding weight, or simply making us feel and look better. Others just enjoy a good workout, as reflected in the utilitarian approach taken by an investment officer from Newport Beach, California: "To me, yoga is great physical training, not something spiritual or religious. I want to be as effective as I can in my job. It's results-driven."[4] However, yoga's deeper benefit is tied to releasing expectations of outcome while resting our awareness—our minds—in our bodies.

## Today's Yoga Scene

Whatever the reason for its immense popularity, yoga is no longer reserved for bendy thirty-somethings with money to spare, or for yogi adepts living in *ashrams* (Hindu spiritual communities). People are coming to yoga with injuries and disabilities, while no doubt many are attracted to that "yoga high," or the feeling at the end of an asana session—smiling, perspiring, and slightly flushed. Others continue to find in yoga a source of wisdom from which to understand their lives and our world. While more men are practicing, young and middle-aged women remain its main practitioners.

As yoga's popularity has grown, so have practitioners' preferences in style. Shopping on the local yoga marketplace has never been better, as consumers gravitate to what they like most, including the latest in practice styles. There is hot yoga; precision yoga, a yoga of flow and endurance; gentle yoga; meditative yoga; and a yoga of energy mastery. There is something for almost everyone's tastes. And it is a buyer's market. As in other industries, broad availability has led to over-saturation in some places. In a two-mile radius of one large Midwestern city, there are eight separate sites where yoga is taught.

While yoga's status as a great fitness workout has helped expand awareness and increase classes and practitioners, its popularity has also turned heads in the medical establishment.[5] Since the growth of wellness alternatives can mean that dollars flow outside of conventional medicine, many hospitals, clinics, medical training programs, and research centers now explore and promote yoga's efficacy as complementary to such care. With attention drawn to its potency, yoga becomes more valued as a tool for addressing specific conditions like asthma or back problems. Complementing mainstream care may be the natural progression of an alternative modality as physicians are more apt to refer patients to classes. Other observers see this development as co-optation, stripping yoga of its philosophical roots as a holistic lifestyle.

Bookstore shelves reveal much about the current state of American yoga.[6] There are how-to books, calendars, tapes, and CDs, including those produced by the industry giant, *Yoga Journal.* Specialized Hatha yoga books provide twenty-eight-day exercise plans targeting specific types of students and health conditions. There are books for the chic (*Yoga Chick: A Hip Guide to Everything Om* and *Cool Yoga Tricks*; and the geek: *Yoga for Wimps* and *Yoga for Regular Guys: The Best Damn Workout on the Planet*). Recent publications have provocative titles blending the fitness and wellness motifs (*Yoga Fights Flab: A 30-Day Program to Tone, Trim, and Flatten Your Trouble Spots*; *Yoga Abs: Moving From Your Core*; and *Yoga for Healthy Knees: What You Need for Pain Prevention and Rehabilitation*). Others tailor to those in special life situations or with special needs:

pregnancy, airline travel, and better sleep. Although most books address the physical aspects, many also address yoga as a multifaceted spiritual discipline.

## Spiritual Origins

Yoga's social reality—whether on a bookstore shelf or on the mat—reflects the meeting of an ancient Indian spiritual path and American commercialism. Recently lost in the glitter is the fact that yoga as a holistic discipline long preceded its status as great exercise or therapeutic rehabilitation. The degree to which personal transformation (*parinama*) is made a centerpiece in yoga classes varies greatly with the type of yoga being taught.

The story of yoga in America began in the late 1800s under the influence of the Theosophical Society and its sponsorship of Indian teachers.[7] Sri Ramakrishna was a great Indian master of *Bhakti Yoga* where love and devotion is central to *sayujya*—union with the Lord, or Absolute Truth. Sri Ramakrishna's student, Swami Vivekananda, embodied the complementary paths of *Jnana* and *Raja Yoga*, where discriminating wisdom and meditation are harnessed to realize Absolute Truth, as manifested in union with our True Self. Neither man would have associated the term "yoga" solely with practicing physical poses but rather with its root meaning as unifying with what is absolute, ultimate, or divine.

Vivekananda attended the first World Parliament of Religions in Chicago in 1893 and became an instant sensation and source of great curiosity, presenting yoga's tenets and practical roadmap as embodied in Hindu thought. His approach linked modern science—from physics to psychology to medicine—with the experiences and insights of yogis. The result was a convergence of Eastern philosophical teachings and Western scientific notions—a precursor to New Age thought—that Americans received as their first taste of how transformation was possible through *sadhana*, or practice. Yoga became known as an exotic path to peace and happiness, where attaining *moksha* meant overcoming the attachment to an illusory view of things which obscures our true nature.

By the 1930s, the mystic Paramahansa Yogananda attracted the curious, the offbeat, and the occasional philanthropist-devotee with his meditative approach to yoga. Followers built an ashram in the Los Angeles area as his (and yoga's) popularity grew with establishment of his Self-Realization Fellowship and its publishing house. A decade later, Indra Devi arrived in Southern California and taught Hollywood celebrities. By the 1950s, Walt and Magana Baptiste had started teaching yoga in San Francisco. However, except for contortionist and mind-over-matter exhibitions for those attracted to sensationalism, national recognition would not fully happen until the cultural revolution of the 1960s.

Yogic spirituality surfaced in the late 1960s and 1970s among thousands of young adults following Indian teachers. The Beatles and other British rock stars were the initial role models. Swami Rama, Swami Muktananada, Maharishi Mahesh Yogi, Sai Baba, Sri Prabhupad, Meher Baba, Yogi Bhajan, Amrit Desai, and Maharaj Ji became the gateways to Eastern ideas for younger Americans. As the hippie counterculture, with its emphasis on consciousness expansion, morphed into New Age culture, yoga eventually spread to college-educated, liberal, and health-conscious females. Spiritually inclined classes became, and often remain, an eclectic mix of philosophy and meditation, poses and breathwork, and chanting and visualization.

In twenty-first century America, spiritual yoga draws from different and not entirely congruent wellsprings of ancient philosophical inspiration. Many retreat centers and ashrams provide Hatha yoga along with teachings from the *Samkhya*, Classical Yoga, and *Vedanta* traditions. These are major Hindu philosophical schools, or *darshanas*, acknowledging the authority of the ancient scriptures or *Vedas*. Teachings of the Samkhya school provide a cosmic worldview of the interplay of Matter and Consciousness. Classical Yoga relies on Samkhya understandings in outlining a roadmap for personal liberation from suffering through specific disciplines, including those laid out by the great sage Patanjali in *The Yoga Sutra*. Perhaps most influential is Vedanta, drawing from the mystically inspired Upanishads to address the nature of reality and of oneself. Some yoga retreat centers also incorporate the *Tantric* elements of *Shaivism*, exploring how the principle of *Shiva*, or formless, supreme consciousness, offers reconnection with our inner divinity through unity with potent *Shakti* energy. Still other centers offer a uniquely blended version of these teachings.

Whichever philosophies inspire it, Yoga as a spiritual path, or *marga*, includes practices that lead us to awareness of our true nature by opening and unifying body, mind, and heart. Postures open the body while drawing attention to movement and energy through the breath. Meditation turns attention further inward, quieting the mind and opening us to our inherent wisdom. Chanting uses repetition of sacred syllables to open the heart to the frequency of love. These coordinated practices (and others) balance our subtle energy, allowing for deeper transformation. When practiced as part of a larger community, yoga has the potential to further affect our world through positive intention and selfless service.

On a superficial level, separating spiritual yoga today from an exclusively fitness-oriented or health-oriented yoga seems quite understandable. Yoga's spiritual aim appears distant from the intentions of most students. More deeply, its esoteric geography of the body, with energy channels or *nadis* and energy centers known as *chakras*, does not translate easily into mainstream medicine's research protocols, nor does it resonate as readily with the fitness scene. Equally difficult to comprehend for many is yoga's claim that a universal energy-consciousness pervades everything in the universe. Despite different understandings and priorities for practice, yoga attracts all those who seek greater balance in their lives.

Yoga begins by gently inviting each student to look within, to open the body, and to synchronize movement with the breath. Its promise of transformation is fueled by finding and maintaining balance—physically, mentally, emotionally, and spiritually. On the face of it, yoga does not require belief in any doctrines to have this effect, only openness to one's experience. In the hands of a gifted teacher, however, the common rituals of a Hatha yoga class anchored by philosophical teachings help to support the transformative process. And since our well-being requires balance wherever and however we practice—no matter how superficially—perhaps this intrinsic human need is yet another reason yoga's popularity has grown in America. By its very nature, yoga is an accessible, practical, and easy-to-understand way to become more centered and to feel truly happy.

Yoga, then, is our gateway for returning to the innate human condition—at peace with ourselves and our world, with flexibility of mind and body and heart. As such, even the most physical or materialistic forms are treated here as yoga, to the possible disappointment of purists. After all, yoga's root meaning—"to join or unify"—refers equally to coordinating mind and movement through the breath in the *vinyasa*, or flow workout, as it does to the profound accomplishment of dissolving the lower mind while resting in our true nature.

## Centering on American Practice

This book addresses yoga's uniquely American journey—taking something ancient and holistic, creating a very contemporary practice, and witnessing its effects on both the society and the discipline. Yoga's recent and prominent growth appears to poke holes in any stereotypical image of America as unsophisticated, xenophobic, and intolerant, suspicious of that which is foreign-born. Rather, yoga's growth seems to contribute to a depiction of the country as more open-minded, embracing diversity and what is best of the exotic while transforming it into something its own. Integration of the foreign has been among the country's highest ideals. Yoga's prominence in certain geographic areas and its invisibility in others may be evidence of its attractiveness to the more tolerant, cosmopolitan, and open-armed among us.

This book is divided into three broad sections that depict a seamless, interrelated web called "American yoga"—the context for practice and the vehicle by which ordinary people gain insight into their lives. The chapters run from the more social and conceptual to the highly personal and heartfelt. Each can be read separately as well as part of the larger whole, much like yoga practice—alone while with others.

The first section, "Transforming Yoga," looks at the yoga scene today and includes the insights and perspectives of those involved in its development. Here, we explore yoga as a social phenomenon, identifying practical implications of the changes it is undergoing and what it must not lose—its transformative potential through practice.

The second section, entitled "Teachers, Teachings, and Transformation," introduces concepts and principles that tie our physical experience of yoga practice to a deeper understanding of the path. We explore how well-being, higher consciousness, and love are all part of the yogic path of transformation. They make us feel more fully alive and are among the many gifts that both teachers and students experience.

The third section of the book—"Transforming Self"—is a testament to yoga's enduring role in igniting and nurturing personal change in practitioners. Drawing upon their experiences, we find how such metamorphosis manifests and triggers subtle insight and dramatic turnarounds. Here, too, we find yoga's tangible effects, by taking classes and through activities "away from the mat" when we are in unfamiliar physical, emotional, or intellectual territory. Outside our habitual comfort zones, we are forced to reflect on the meaning of who we are and what we do and on how yoga promotes such self-reflection and study.

It seems these three sections reflect the more important and interrelated parts of my own life—the first as a trained observer of the social scene, the second as a certified yoga instructor, and the third as a student who has been challenged to apply yoga's teachings to life. To aid the reader in reflecting on the role of yoga in her life, I have included a series of questions in appendix B to be entertained after reading each chapter. It is my conviction that the greater attention that we can give to yoga's transformation in America and its potent role in our lives, the more likely its gifts to humankind will be preserved. I hope that this book contributes to yoga's efficacy as a path leading to authentic happiness, in fulfillment of Tirumalai Krishnamacharya's claim that it is "India's greatest gift to the world," including our small part of it.[8]

# *Part 1*

# Transforming Yoga

*This first section of the book highlights the current state of yoga practice in America, its interplay with the environment, and how and why its transformation occurred. Chapters focus on the nature of a yoga subculture, affected by growth of a multibillion-dollar industry, and its attractiveness to the medical establishment. Readers are exposed to the human side of this development, reflected in the words of those contributing to yoga's transformation at retreat centers and yoga studios while riding this tidal wave of change and confronting the ethical issues and financial opportunities it presents. Here, too, the reader is introduced to Hatha yoga's cousin—melodious chanting—which is undergoing a similar transformation.*

*In the end, we might ask how well yoga's original gift is maintained in the face of it all, and what will be necessary to assure that one's own practice embodies yoga's promise as a source of guidance and inspiration. Only by exploring the current challenge can practitioners find balanced solutions, perhaps somewhere between the extremes that beckon them as they search for the deeper meaning of their lives.*

CHAPTER ONE

# Yoga Class, Culture Clash

"That strap really helped me, and the teacher's assist released tension in my shoulders." "I didn't like her approach, and I hated the background music." "My mind was focused in class, yet completely relaxed." "I appreciated his discussion of yoga philosophy." These feelings, attitudes, and judgments reflect the existence of a yoga subculture—a shared knowledge among its *yogis* and *yoginis* (male and female practitioners) that forms a unique part of American life. In this subculture, one finds unfamiliar movements and exotic gestures, shared terms of subtlety and grace, ritual sights and sounds, and people and places to which we are relating in growing numbers. Feeling a part of this legacy—and solidarity with other students—depends on our commitment to yoga and the extent to which we consider it a central part of our lives.

In *A History of Modern Yoga*, British historian Elisabeth De Michelis describes the contemporary yoga experience this way:

> The actual classroom may be a gym, or community centre hall or the more soothing atmosphere of a yoga centre or a teacher's

> living room. There may be an introductory and/or final short reading or theoretical 'instructions'; different styles of yoga will be characterized by a slower or faster pace, or different paces will be found across various sessions of the same style of yoga; some styles of yoga or sessions will be run with a greater sense of 'social' or 'communal' event, others will emphasize inwardness and quiet individual work, etc.—but the overall structure remains the same.[1]

Despite variation in content and style, almost all classes share, on some level, in Indian terminology and beliefs. They also share physical artifacts, like clothing, music, belts, mats, and blocks. Most students observe the same class norms about not staring, talking, or touching. And no doubt many have had that shared experience of release, frustration, and laughter at an unplanned landing on their sitz bones.

A traditional yoga class in America includes an identifiable ritual order. A centering phase with relaxed mind and felt-separation from our everyday life leads into an active phase of asana practice (ideally with breath awareness). A cooling-down follows, with a final phase of rest and relaxation. Then, there is that resulting sense of rejuvenation or feeling of exhaustion. From a yogic perspective, these stages mirror, in microcosm, the wider phases of our lives—birth and awakening; activity through concentration, effort, and determination; decline and eventual death; only to be followed by our rebirth into the world. In one sense, yoga class is our continuous dress rehearsal in the art of living and dying.

Despite this broadly shared classroom experience, yoga's rapid growth yields a range of class offerings, approaches taken by teachers from different backgrounds, and widening student expectations about what yoga should be. Yoga's greater popularity means we are often taking classes for overlapping reasons, and yoga's subculture has shifted in character and splintered into segments. Maybe this has always been the case with yoga, but now it is easier to distinguish the three broadest motivations for practicing—to get a good physical workout as a form of fitness, to promote our health or healing, and to follow a deeper transformative path. There are now fitness yogis, health and healing yogis, spiritual yogis, and all possible combinations. Some of us practice for all three reasons.

## Making Room

Beth, Ross, and Amber appear to be the typical middle-class suburban Chicago family, yet they are less than average in one glaring sense: they all practice yoga. Beth is in her forties, a school teacher and follower since the 1980s of Gurumayi (also known as Swami Chidvilasananda), leader of Siddha Yoga at the Shree Muktananada Ashram in South Fallsburg, New York. She practices Hatha yoga postures daily as part of her spiritual path, which also includes a session with pranayama, chanting, and meditation. Every other year, she travels to the ashram from her Midwestern home. The term "spirituality" for Beth does not mean exclusive adherence to doctrine and faith as much as it entails exploring her shared humanity through experiential practices that open the body, mind, and heart to a deeper understanding of life and one's place in the wider world.

Beth's husband Ross is a contractor who respects her holistic lifestyle and recently began taking a restorative yoga class after surgery for a work-related injury to his rotator cuff. Amber, their on-the-go teenage daughter, became a vegetarian a few years ago for health reasons and because of a love of animals. She has no interest in yoga's spiritual side—the breathwork, ethical precepts, meditation, and metaphysical teachings. For her, yoga is merely a good fitness workout that her mother pays for weekly at a local wellness center.

This Midwestern family typifies the diversity found in yoga classes today. Those motivated largely by deeper transformative concerns are likely to differ in outlook, expectation, and training from those attracted to yoga as a fitness workout or therapeutic rehabilitation. In other words, segments among the yoga subculture are looking for slightly different things from yoga. With the growing number of secular teachers and students entering the market, the subculture as a whole is being transformed. This transformation is reflected at yoga retreats and conferences, in teacher training programs, at chanting sessions, and wherever else its members gather.

**A student census conducted among ninety-four students at an urban Midwestern wellness center found the following reasons for practicing yoga:**

| | |
|---|---|
| **Keep fit/Get in shape** | 77% |
| **Deal with stress or a health condition** | **73%** |
| Work with a specific teacher/yoga style | 73% |
| Become more centered | 65% |
| How I feel afterward | 54% |
| Convenient days and times | 54% |
| Convenient location | 50% |
| **Spiritual outlook or practice** | **35%** |
| Challenge myself | 35% |

Some students fall cleanly into one of three broad and interrelated practitioner segments—fitness yoga, health and healing yoga, or spiritual yoga—while others do not (see figure 1). With time, students may evolve to integrate more of these reasons for practicing, yet their differences might just point to certain subtle tensions in the yoga subculture today. If you practice Hatha yoga, ask yourself: At the beginning and end of a class, do you like to chant "Om" (that primordial sound of the energetic universe from which everything manifests)? Do you like a rock or jazz background, *kirtan* chants, or silence? Do you prefer detailed description of musculature and movement, or is minimal wording best? Are assists important to you? Do you have a regular meditation practice to complement your asanas? Is strengthening, toning, or healing a goal? Do you prefer a loving, supportive teacher or a more impersonal, rigorous instructor? (See the practitioner quiz in appendix A).

**Figure 1. Overlapping Reasons for Practice**

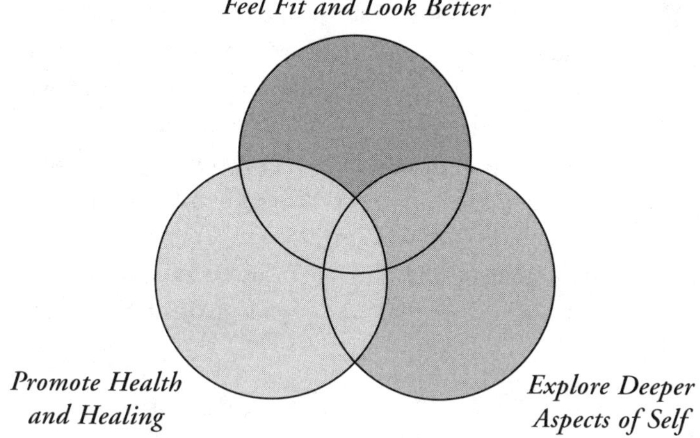


## Diversifying Style and Motivation

While many factors have contributed to yoga's recent popularity, an interest in fitness has dramatically expanded yoga's overall visibility and probably accounts for the majority practicing one of its many forms. Consequently, yoga is common fare in community, recreation, and fitness centers nationwide. In times of greater economic prosperity, the public has become predisposed to practice in greater numbers, and they have done so by the millions.

The popularity of fitness-oriented styles has had a profound influence on contemporary American yoga, reflected in the assessment by Georg Feuerstein, the Western world's esteemed yoga scholar: Yoga's deep philosophical and spiritual foundations are rarely understood by teachers and students, as yoga is "widely reduced to gymnastics and fitness training, without any reference to, or experience of, the kundalini and higher forms of consciousness, never mind the great ideal of spiritual liberation."[2]

Srivatsa Ramaswami, a yogi in the tradition of the great Krishnamacharya, argues that

> What you might call Western or American yoga has taken on a distinctive character. Yoga, with its unique approach to physical culture, has to compete with other popular forms of exercise, like gym workouts or even gymnastics. We have 'power yoga' and other similar systems in which considerable exertion is used, like the pumping and jumping in *Ashtanga* yoga vinyasas á la gymnastic floor exercises. Though these were part of the ancient vinyasa yoga, several parameters such as breathing requirements, keeping the heart rate and breath rate under check, have been passed over in favor of generating excitement.[3]

Amber's fitness yoga, while often very physically demanding, is less personally challenging than the yoga practiced by her mother as a lifestyle commitment and as part of an ashram. In other words, one can leave the fitness yoga subculture at the recreation center door, while yoga as a lifestyle affects everything—from diet and moral conduct to outlook and methods for seeking greater balance, or even liberation, in this life.

Health professionals have begun treating yoga as a complementary healing modality. When coupled with the popular fitness craze, their interest has led to greater acceptance of yoga's role in treatment and prevention. This acceptance has birthed another subcultural segment—health and healing yoga. Historian De Michelis argues that "except in cases of thoroughly utilitarian (fitness or recreational) performance . . . some notion of healing and personal growth is likely to provide the deepest rationale for practice."[4] Yoga's capacity to heal and promote health has broad interest among those holding different views of the physical body. Its healing role motivates Americans who follow the Western medical model as well as those who treat physical conditions holistically, as a function of a subtle energetic relationship between body, mind, emotion, and spirit. The latter approach blends well with yoga's transformative role as a form of spirituality and as an entryway for exploring ourselves more deeply.

As physicians and mental health therapists have become involved with healing alternatives like yoga in their personal lives, they also have begun referring patients like Ross to classes in growing numbers. While yoga complements mainstream medicine, it is experiencing a secular double-effect: It is being reduced to its physicality, while mainstream medicine subjects the more physical side of yoga to rigorous scientific and clinical investigations.

One measure of whether a yoga class falls more within the fitness and health categories or within a deeper transformative one may well be whether breath work is given serious attention. As Feuerstein has put it, "breath control equals mental control" in yoga practice.[5] Where we are taught to place our attention in class and whether we learn and practice breath work determines if we are able to work directly with prana, the breath's inner correspondence to our more subtle energy. Pranayama is a "threshold practice" to yoga's deeper side.

## Spiritual Yoga

While the physical emphases in both fitness-and health-oriented yoga reinforce each other, both types emerged from yoga as a holistic discipline and lifestyle. This subcultural segment preserves the path's essential meaning—the art of living fully—while feeding and being fed by the mainstream. New Age culture played a significant role in incubating yoga spirituality in the 1970s and 1980s. Even as the hippie counterculture faded as a movement, the concern for things natural to eat, wear, and revere became a common part of lifestyles in college towns and hipper, youthful sections of large cities. Natural food stores and restaurants, New Age bookstores, gem shops, natural healing centers, co-ops, temples, churches, and other establishments proliferated. An alternative spiritual press preserved awareness of yoga's transformative side and its ultimate goal of Self-realization.

Yoga began its slow evolution from alternative to complementary health practice at about this same time, as popular movements espousing optimal well-being embraced Eastern thought. Yoga remained part of the spiritual palette for those in the New Age following Asian gurus and Western psychotherapists, as well as for those branching out to create new yoga styles. Breath work, once reserved as an integral part of yoga practice, emerged as its own healing modality.

As the fitness frenzy captured popular attention by the new millennium, spiritually committed practitioners who still applied yoga's essential teachings to their daily lives became a less visible and prominent part of the yoga scene. Ramaswami describes the change this way: "Only a fraction of the people are really interested in studying yoga in its original version."[6] Gifted teachers of yoga's ancient traditions appear even harder to find than students, since "living yoga" demands a strong commitment to mind training and serious self-study while showing little interest in treating yoga merely as a workout, body strengthener, or rehabilitator (as valuable as they may be).

As yoga has slowly become a part of the modern health and fitness, fee-for-service industry, yoga teachers are required to speak the language of Western medicine (at least anatomy and physiology), more than they are of ancient Indian philosophical concepts. As a result, Ramaswami asserts, "many of the lofty and subtle principles of the older yoga system are being lost."[7] Serious study of ancient yogic physiology and diagnostic and curative methods remains largely unintegrated with the dominant Western medical paradigm. In turn, this lack of integration creates a Western yoga different from the more traditional yoga practice in India which, according to author Marina Budhos, tends to be "longer and devote more time to mindful breathing and meditation."[8] And as Feuerstein noted, the subtle and deeper energetic dimension is often lost in the process.

Given these developments, America's diverse yoga subculture may be a symptom of a deeper issue. While different segments of America's new yoga family are often embodied in the very same teacher, student, or family, yoga as a social phenomenon is morphing into something fundamentally at variance with what it was meant to be.

## Losing Yoga's Deeper Meaning

Millions of us attend classes each week because we enjoy what yoga has to offer. We may not think about the larger issue of what is happening to yoga, nor are we likely to consider this issue very important in the context of our daily lives—getting kids off to school, engaging in work, or relaxing and going out with friends. In short, yoga may be our hour-and-a-half "asana oasis" from that busy life. What we experience through yoga and what we enjoy about it may seem to have little to do with the broader issues of the wider world or the more personal concerns of our day.

However, the larger picture of contemporary yoga suggests that social forces beyond our control—media appetite for entertainment, population shifts around us, economics of the fitness industry, ubiquitous star-gazing in pop culture, developments in the medical profession, or influences on the fringe of our culture—can subtly affect our personal experience of yoga. While practicing makes us feel good and heals us in many ways seemingly independent of these influences, yoga's transformational work depends directly on how deeply we wish to travel down its ancient pathway. The deeper we travel, the more likely we are to confront the barriers and obstacles—the knots—that hold us back from releasing into who we truly are or what we can ultimately become. The deeper we journey, the more likely we are to fully accept and make friends with ourselves—to release the willful struggle of mind over body and to experience the bliss and happiness attending to the path.

At the other end of the spectrum is the shallow understanding of yoga spirituality which feeds the nonpracticing public's stereotyped image of it and is offensive to those who view the path as a way to explore themselves more deeply. While yoga spirituality is irrelevant to those who do not relate at all to its deeper message, shallowness leads to cynicism about yoga's essential meaning as a holistic discipline and way of life. Even those who practice for fitness reasons are beginning to suspect that there is something amiss, reflected in the disturbing yet insightful observation by NBC Nightly News' Clare Duffy:

> Yoga—it's a way to feel slightly better about really a very self-absorbed pastime—i.e., working out at a gym and checking yourself out in the mirror. It gets grafted on with this sense of 'Oh, I'm at one with the universe and the inner light in me goes with you.' Is it really spiritual? I don't know. In some ways it's just a way to feel a little better about our essential self-absorption and not more than that.[9]

If this is what yoga has become for many American practitioners, then it is truly in a state of crisis. It is akin to celebrating Christmas without its essential meaning in mind and feeling lost under an avalanche of consumer gift-giving and self-interested concern for what we receive from it. Rather than reinforcing self-centeredness, yoga should be essentially the opposite—a process for dropping our self-absorption to live more fully in each moment and in the service of others. The extent to which Americans in general and practitioners in particular do not hold to such an outlook on yoga is the single best indicator of how far yoga has strayed from its original meaning.

How then can yoga as transformative experience remain a viable, visible option for practitioners as its subculture spreads, diversifies, and becomes associated with a fitness regimen? One measure of yoga's continued effectiveness is the very tangible benefit of well-being experienced by its students. However, if living in the moment, loosening opinion, addressing negativity, and opening the tender heart are not addressed by the growing number of teachers, yoga might only be seducing us, while it is being reduced to a physical workout. The millions turning to it today will not fully recognize yoga's power to transform them into wiser, more centered and compassionate beings while inducing in them a deeper awareness of higher states of being where the potential lies as well for transforming the world around them.

How did American yoga get to this crisis point—more of a weekly workout than a doorway to deeper understandings?

CHAPTER 2 TWO

# An American Revolution

*Popularity becomes a curse.*
*Popularity introduces dilution.*
—Geeta Iyengar

For clear evidence of how yoga is changing in America, look no further than *Yoga Journal.* For its thirtieth anniversary issue, which appeared in October 2005, this venerable American yoga bible ran a cover article entitled "Why America Loves Yoga and How It's Changing Lives," about yoga's spread to the mainstream. Committed teachers from small towns across the country were introducing yoga to farmers, fishermen, ministers, and ranchers—people from all walks of life who were learning yoga's benefits as an anchor for a more centered life and a refuge from stress or chronic pain.

Another article in that issue prognosticated about yoga's future—that yoga might more fully spread throughout society and into the very halls of power through business franchising, medical expansion, institutionalized higher learning, and mainstream media programming. "So we don't really expect yoga to have totally conquered and colonized every aspect of American life by 2030," the writer mused. "But it may indeed play a much larger role in our culture than it does today." But *which* yoga will play that role—the yoga of the fitness crowd, the yoga practiced by those following holistic teachings, the therapeutic yoga at wellness centers, or all three forms as one and the same path?

## Roots and Growth

When *Yoga Journal* was established in the mid-1970s, there was already enough impetus to support a national magazine dedicated to the discipline.[1] A number of college-educated young adults, buoyed by their growing interest in meditation and yoga, already entertained values considered countercultural in the 1960s—self-care, vegetarianism, natural healing, and psycho-spiritual growth. Gurus from India, Tibet, Japan, Vietnam and Korea had been invited to the United States by their American followers. Ashrams and yoga and meditation centers sprang up in cities along both coasts, and retreat centers were established in the Rockies and Appalachians. Notable early examples of these centers were Yogi Bhajan's Healthy, Happy, Holy Organization, founded in 1969, and the Bikram Yoga College, founded in 1974. Urban centers of international organizations—like the Divine Light Mission—spread throughout the country and authors taking up the Eastern trail, like Ram Dass (Dr. Richard Alpert), became familiar names. Practicing asanas and experiencing their health benefits happened within a wider spiritual context. By the 1980s, an emerging New Age culture provided the rationale, worldview, products, and services to meet practitioners' needs at bookshops, retreat centers, natural food stores, vegetarian restaurants, churches, and holistic health clinics.

Popular yoga figures already included B. K. S. Iyengar, author of the classic *Light on Yoga*, as well as others trained by Krishnamacharya in India[2]—K. Patabhi Jois, Indra Devi, and K. T. V.

Desikachar, among them. Krishnamacharya had treated asana and pranayama as aspects of meditation while refining them as physical practices. Iyengar and his family members would continue to teach thousands of yoga instructors over the succeeding decades in systematic refinements of asana practice, its healing benefits, and the requirements of living a yogic lifestyle. With time, a network of official Iyengar centers sprouted, as did studios for Patabhi Jois's Ashtanga yoga and Desikachar's Viniyoga. Those trained by Swami Sivananda in India included Swami Satchidananda and Swami Vishnudevananda, whose Integral Yoga and Sivananda Yoga centers, respectively, also dotted North America.

By the early 1990s, Beryl Bender Birch in New York and Bryan Kest in California had developed "power yoga" as a Westernized version of Ashtanga. "People began to see yoga as a way to work out" and power yoga, as Ann Pizer pointed out, "brought yoga into the gyms of America."[3] As a result, yoga classes were clearly diversifying into varied styles, with some more physically rigorous and demanding than others. The added rigor did not necessarily equate to shallow spirituality, unless the focus became essentially gymnastic.

Three parallel trends contributed to the mainstream's growing embrace of yoga throughout the 1990s and to growth in readership for yoga magazines. *First, greater social acceptance of yoga would require openness to experimentation.* Social movements questioning traditional roles had already succeeded in gaining greater public acceptance by stretching our sense of what constituted normal gender behavior at home and at play. By 1990, lifestyle and role experimentation had become socially acceptable among liberal constituencies in the country, and that trend continues. Many in the middle class opted for more egalitarian and androgynous roles as the image of a yoga student slowly embraced stereotypical attributes associated with traditional femininity (gentleness, receptivity, and flexibility) and masculinity (endurance, strength, and control).

*Second, experimenting role models who could generate interest, excitement, and empathy among the public had to receive mainstream media attention.* Movies and television programs—especially the daytime "tell-all talk" of The Phil Donahue Show, The Oprah Winfrey show, and a host of others—showcased the sharing of personal information with the public (This trend continues with the advent of blog Web sites and podcasting). These forms of entertainment served as a continuous outlet for starlets, star-wannabes, the famous, and the not-so-famous to publicly share androgynous lifestyles and alternative practices.

The entertainment industry's tell-all celebrity stories eventually spread everywhere—on television and radio, in magazines and movies, and eventually on the Web. They covered entertaining topics of interest to largely female audiences. Yoga was one of these topics. A legion of experimenting stars added their names to a growing list of famous practitioners touting the many health and fitness benefits of a now more rigorous yoga: Madonna, Sting, Cindy Crawford, Helen Hunt, Christy Turlington, Gwyneth Paltrow, Reese Witherspoon, Kareem Abdul-Jabbar, Barry Zito, Eddie George, Sandra Day O'Connor, Julia Louis-Dreyfuss, Jane Fonda, Angelina Jolie, Sarah Jessica Parker, and Charlie Sheen. Nationally renowned physicians Andrew Weil and Dean Ornish joined the fray. A few celebrities stressed yoga's deeper message as the list grew almost overnight. Yet spiritual commentary fell on mostly deaf ears. As a Pew Research Center survey found, generations succeeding the baby boomers (tagged as Generation X and Generation Next) are more materialistic and less concerned with spirituality than are earlier generations; yoga could shift to follow suit and easily attract these younger generations.[4]

Key to this shift was the evolving message of pop culture stardom from "idolize me to emulate me." Writing for the *Los Angeles Times* about the media influence of today's glamorous people, film critic Carina Chocano concluded that stars "may appear in TV shows that aren't so much TV shows as a chance to observe celebrities in their natural habitats. Which kind of resemble ours. Mainstream magazines have transformed themselves from facilitators of idol worship to guides of glamour consumption."[5] Many adults apparently got their first faddish taste of yoga as friends, family members, and co-workers followed celebrities to class.

*Third, growing interest in yoga would require an energetic outlook and socially respectable outlets.* Emphasizing the benefits of getting in shape, feeling fit, and enjoying life more fully, the fitness industry used medical information to encourage a growing market through the franchising of fitness centers, the proliferation of community recreation centers and spas, and the spread of personalized training. The industry expanded exponentially with the aging of baby boomers but also attracted younger generations. "Stress reduction," much like weight reduction, became a catchphrase in the face of new and stressful technological changes. At the same time, the popular media used health, beauty, and self-care tips to hook viewers and readers in an ever more image-conscious society.

Eventually, this workout perspective began to influence Hatha yoga teaching and to infiltrate a growing yoga market. Ramaswami puts it this way: People wanting dynamic exercises found "the old yoga a bit too sedate. So these energetic exercises have drawn a number of enthusiasts to yoga. Furthermore, many Westerners like to 'sweat it out.' So systems of yoga where one is made to profusely sweat by artificially altering the ambient temperature have also become popular."[6] Lifestyle openness and experimentation soon converged with widespread messages about fitness, beauty, stress, and relaxation, first on the coasts and then elsewhere.

In turn, these three broad currents cross-fertilized the growing mainstream interest in what were once exclusively "New Age" concepts: natural healing products, holistic health modalities, comparative spirituality, and edgy science. Thoughtful writers such as Deepak Chopra, Charles Tart, and Ken Wilber brought together Eastern thought and Western science, as Swami Vivekananda had done a century earlier. Drs. Weil, Ornish, and a cadre of physicians with one foot outside the medical establishment touted the benefits of natural healing alternatives, including a now-evolving yoga practiced without a deep spiritual message in mind.

The public took heed of yoga's healing power, and mainstream medicine assessed its efficacy. Harvard physician David Eisenberg noted the sharp rise throughout the 1990s in the use of alternative therapies like yoga.[7] To the tune of $12.2 billion in out-of-pocket payments annually, the public increasingly turned to such services and dietary supplements. At the same time, some medical training programs and hospitals began to teach alternative models of healing alongside mainstream medicine. By 1998, Congress established the National Center for Alternative and Complementary Medicine (NCACM) as part of the National Institutes of Health in Bethesda, Maryland. As the Office of Alternative Medicine (OAM) within the Center began to fund Hatha yoga studies, the American Medical Association and its publication arm, the *Journal of the American Medical Association* (*JAMA*), also sought to publish research on Hatha yoga, acupuncture, ginseng, faith-based practices, and other alternative topics. Other mainstream medical journals followed their lead.

The result was a compelling paradigm of cutting-edge thinking and research findings, a growing market for natural healing products and wellness practices, and a committed readership for a host of holistic health publications. *Yoga Journal* editor Ann Cushman experienced firsthand the rapid expansion of the yoga industry in America and these congealing forces by the new millennium:

> Everyone wants New Age talent, products, and services. 'Nightline,' '20/20,' daytime talk shows, as well as cable and radio are scrambling for good New Age talent to appear as guests and consultants. Coffee houses and bookstores are booking New Age entertainment, as well as placing New Age images on their walls, tables, and even coffee mugs. Large chain bookstores like Borders are now having monthly psychic fairs, and even travel agencies are packaging 'intuitive tours' and 'vision quests.'[8]

## The Spread to the Midsection

By 2000, all the dynamite needed to ignite a national yoga explosion was present. With full economic expansion, young and middle-aged professionals had larger expendable incomes. Yoga images were everywhere, from Arm & Hammer ads for toothpaste to Mel Gibson's movie, *What Women Want*. Given the power of electronic media, young and middle-aged females unassociated with the New Age, but following the fads and fashions of the rich or famous, now entered the yoga subculture nationwide. Yoga was a *very* hot item, but it had been largely reduced to asana practice and in many instances secularized as a physical workout commodity, healing modality, and a way to remain centered. Studios sprouted throughout cities and eventually made their way into the rural hinterlands. Yoga training programs popped up almost overnight, and new magazines, CDs, and Web sites joined the bandwagon.

As a testament to yoga's growing popularity, Christian writers expressed concern over the dangers associated with its alleged "objectives and realities." One result of their concern was that if yoga was to be taught in public schools throughout the country, it would have to be melted down to asana practice to make it acceptable to secular school boards and Christian Fundamentalist parents. The "Yoga Ed" program adopted in more than one hundred schools from coast to coast had "stripped every piece of anything that anyone could vaguely construe as spiritual or religious out of the program."[9]

This school-based secularization not only reflects yoga's intrinsic physical and psychological benefits but also the clout of the Christian Right when faced with what it sees as a competitor to its path to the truth (despite all the secular developments affecting yoga). Perhaps looking into a mirror and projecting his own intentions, one Christian writer characterized yoga as "a vital part of the largest missionary program in the world," apparently to convert non-Hindus. Another way that Christian churches confronted "the yoga threat" was reported by *Time* in 2005: Appropriating yoga by replacing Sanskrit mantras with Christian words in renaming asanas, which drew the ire of the Hindu American Foundation as intellectual property theft.[10]

Yoga had arrived as a full-fledged industry. In 2001, yoga became a *Time* cover story, and *Newsweek*'s Josh Ulick exclaimed a year later that "yoga may be here to stay."[11] In the spring of 2003, *US Weekly* would ask, "Has Hollywood's Yoga Obsession Gone Too Far?" while stressing yoga's acknowledged role in improving strength and flexibility.[12] The subculture supporting the industry had clearly diversified into fitness yogis, health and healing yogis, and a smaller segment holding to deeper things.

Gifted Hatha teachers were nationally prominent figures, stars in their own right. Power yoga master Baron Baptiste, who grew up in the California fitness scene, rode the power yoga wave as one of a select group of teachers regularly given top billing at conferences around the country, including those organized and sponsored by *Yoga Journal*. Bikram Choudhury, guru to the wealthy and well-known, unflinchingly advertised his hot yoga practice as "the most exciting, hard-working, effective, amusing, and glamorous yoga class in the world." He was also quoted as saying that teachers, with the exception of himself and those he certified, were "a bunch of clowns."[13] Was this a warning to the yoga industry that the growing cadre of teachers was not being properly trained? By 2006, the North American Studio Alliance (NAMASTA) estimated that the number of teachers—many of them part-time—had ballooned to a staggering 70,000 in the United States and Canada.[14] Master teacher and Tantric practitioner Rod Stryker explained the facts simply: "Teaching yoga has become a business in America. The bigger the class, the more teachers you train, the more money you make."[15]

The trend continues. Top-name teachers like Rodney Yee and Seane Corne regularly pack hotel ballrooms and retreat facilities, promoting books and CDs to long lines of adoring practitioners. *Yoga Journal* has launched week long Caribbean cruises with Yee and Baptiste joining Cyndi Lee, Shiva Rea, and other well-known instructors. National teachers run on travel circuits that match any popular rock band's tour schedule.[16]

However, relatively few instructors offering asana classes today also provide regular meditation sessions or classes in yoga philosophy and psychology. Some well-known instructors like Cyndi Lee keep the meditative quality of focused awareness central to their teaching, as when Lee led five hundred people in poses at a Buddhist retreat with monastic Pema Chödrön. Shiva Rea links activist causes and selfless service with business profits and supports a worldwide gathering to unite the global yoga community. Stephen Cope facilitated conferences on Yoga and Buddhism, exploring their interface through practice and discussion. And sympathetic niche magazines like *The Shambhala Sun* periodically address yoga's complementary roots with Buddhist meditation.

Regardless of any interest in spiritual yoga, statistics bear out the growing popularity of a secularized yoga. American Sports Data, Inc.'s Superstudy reported that participation in yoga and pilates was displacing more traditional exercise, with enormous growth among the younger exercise crowd—a ninety-five percent increase from 1998 to 2002 alone.[17] Seventeen million had taken the leap by 2005, spending billions annually on their yoga workouts. By the summer of that same year, an online health, beauty, and fitness center could publicly comment—apparently without embarrassment—that "while yoga is popular, it is not quite mainstream as yet. However, many people have the misconception that yoga is boring, too quiet, *linked to eastern religions and many other myths*." [Emphasis added.][18] That is, yoga is really a rigorous workout, can be done to a rock beat, is immensely fun, and has little or nothing to do with spirituality. The yoga explosion had been clearly set off with secular dynamite (see figure 2 below).

These developments evoke reaction from those with a deep appreciation for yoga's ancient tradition. Surveying American yoga, Georg Feuerstein lamented in 2003 that "most contemporary schools of Hatha-Yoga ignore prana and pranayama, just as they ignore the mental disciplines and spiritual goals, and instead promote a plethora of physical postures (asana). The emphasis is problematical, as it has led to an unfortunate reductionism and distortion of the traditional yogic heritage."[19]

**Figure 2. Factors Contributing to Yoga's Growth**

Yoga's Practicality, Adaptability & Transformative Power
Medicine's Openness to Hatha Yoga's Efficacy
Growth & Influence of "Metrospirituals"
Business Packaging of Yoga as a Leisure Activity
Health and Fitness Centers Opening to Asana-Based Yoga
Adaptable Yoga Organizations and Teaching Innovators
Stripping Yoga of Its Cultural and Religious Roots
Favorable Economic Conditions and More Expendable Income
Materialist, Media-Conscious Generations
Broad Acceptance of Role Experimentation
The Information Age's Media Explosion
Influence of Pop Culture and Celebrity Lifestyles
The Yoga Explosion

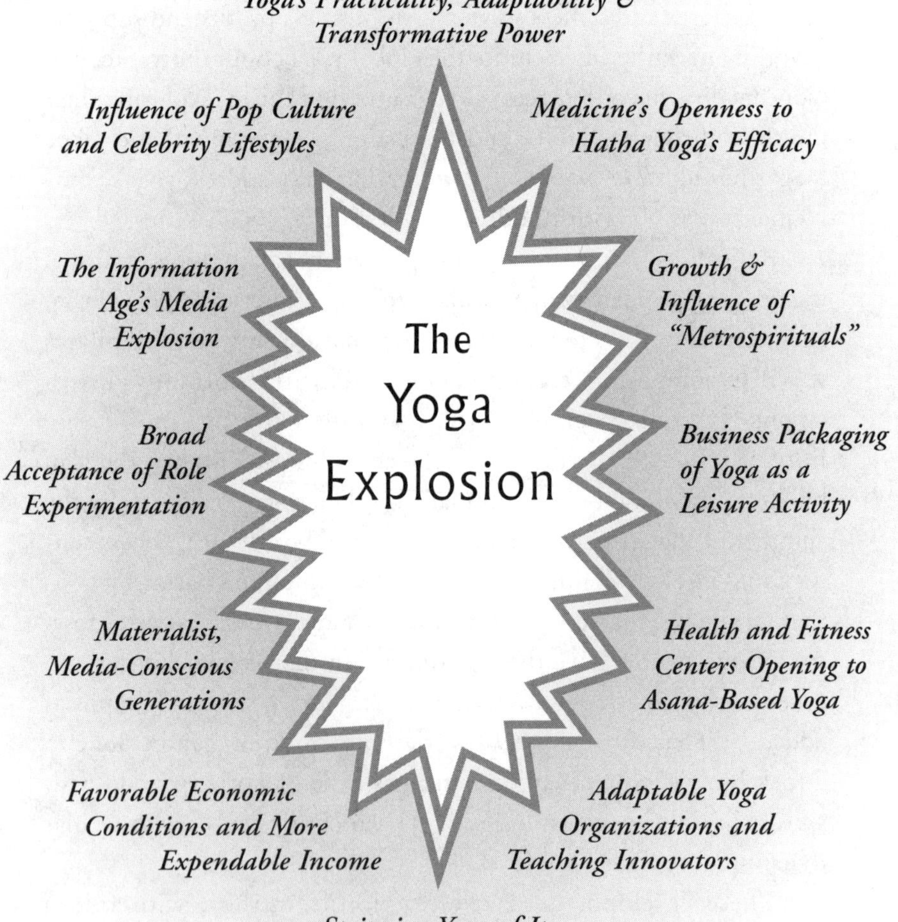

Yet celebration of yoga's diversity and popularity is a more common response to the industry's phenomenal growth, evidenced by editorials in publications of the Yoga Alliance, the International Association of Yoga Therapists, and *Yoga Journal*. Indeed, how difficult it would be *not* to express openness and acceptance, given the consumer and revenue benefits of a path-turned-mainstream industry, much less the professional, community, and educational ramifications of a more fully assimilated activity.

## The View from Ground Zero

Today, that fee-for-service industry is teeming with thousands of teachers providing classes in a variety of locations to millions of students. At ground zero in urban America, yoga is diversified by city, suburb, and neighborhood; classes are provided in virtually every type of living and working space; and instructors offer a variety of traditional forms and hybridized styles. Like other industries before it, yoga is growing unevenly—rapidly in some places while stagnating due to over saturation in others. Such volatility may be natural, with yoga's number of part-time teaching positions offering wages that lead many to supplement their instruction with more sustainable work. After all, a love of asana practice—not a rational assessment of job opportunities—spurred the thousands to train. And that training is further diversified by two hundred-hour and five hundred-hour certification requirements, opportunities at workshops and conferences, and on-the-job apprenticing with seasoned—if not renowned—instructors. Advancements in medical knowledge and technical innovation drive continuous improvements that are eventually shared with teachers.

Many instructors, after years of successful teaching, branch out to open their own studios and confront the challenge of balancing what consumers want with what they know and value about yoga. J. Brown, founder of Brooklyn's Abhyasa Yoga Center, wrote in

2008 of his own challenge at opening a center in an increasingly diversified yoga marketplace: "I've become known as the "breath" guy. . . . Attendance has demonstrated an obvious need and market for an alternative to athletic and ascetic approaches. Assembling a staff for the center has been difficult because I know very few teachers who are working within this framework. In fact, most teachers feel pressured to cater to popular, sometimes injurious, notions."[20]

What is the upshot of yoga's dramatic rise in popularity? While associated largely with asana and spurred by its growth potential, yoga has been stripped down, glamorized, professionalized, and at times disengaged from its historical and cultural roots. Now less attention need be given to yoga as a holistic path of personal purification and freedom, with deep practices that open students to a wider metaphysical worldview and their place in it. If the billions of consumer dollars spent are any indication, most people are apparently satisfied with a narrowly circumscribed yoga. Yet at the same time, a key minority segment has evolved to sustain and carry yoga's deeper message—a segment *Newsweek* writers in the summer of 2006 referred to as "LOHAS," twenty-first century New Agers embodying Lifestyles of Health and Sustainability. A year later, a newly coined term, "metrospirituals," was applied to this same segment.[21]

As American yoga's major media popularizer, *Yoga Journal* best reflects the industry's expansion and promotes its diversification with mainstream credentials. By 2005, the magazine had a paid circulation of 325,000 with a million bimonthly readers. In a press release, its president and CEO John Abbott recognized that the growing statistics on yoga practitioners over the previous ten years meant that "yoga is not a passing fad but a genuine cultural phenomenon and an integral part of the wellness trend in this country."[22] Meanwhile, *Yoga Journal*'s competitors looked to tap into its expanding marketplace. No doubt motivated by spirituality *and* economic realism, in July 2006 editor Deborah Willoughby explained the renaming of her magazine *Yoga International* to *Yoga*

+ *Joyful Living* this way: "Yoga has become so popular that yoga studios are as ubiquitous as Starbucks. This is both interesting as a social phenomenon and useful as a way of introducing more people to the art of applying yogic principles to all aspects of their day-to-day lives: to Joyful Living."[23]

On magazine pages, one finds evidence of how yoga is assimilating into our collective national psyche and interpersonal lives, as well as how its Indian roots are respected but often lost through the forest of its commercial tree branches. Here, too, is clear testimony of yoga's integration into the fabric of the country's institutions as a full-blown industry with educational programming and research enterprises to prove its health benefits, preventive and rehabilitative modalities to ensure its application, and business products and services that expand its profits. It is a measure of *Yoga Journal*'s staying power that advertising dollars not only effectively sell yoga more than thirty years after the magazine's inception in 1975 but also that *Yoga Journal* has become established as a multimillion-dollar, award-winning mainstream publication with an expanding readership base.

The end result of all these developments seems crystal clear: yoga has been easily injected with the nation's penchant for business enterprise. This commercialization is something that yoga's deeper practices are fortunately spared, since it may be too difficult to sell long periods of sitting meditation to watch the turning of one's own mind or the practice of disciplined breath work that moves energy up and down subtle channels of the energy body. Such practices are definitely not as enticing nor as easily promoted as yoga's outer layer—the poses and the products that cater to pre- and post-asana practice by a wide range of businesses and advertisers, educational and health care organizations, and media and entertainment outlets.

A closer look at *Yoga Journal*'s thirtieth anniversary issue exposes the commercialized state of twenty-first-century yoga. This is not a criticism of the magazine but recognition of the "facts of life" dictated by the publication business. Two-thirds of *Yoga Journal*'s 168 pages are filled with advertising falling into seven categories: natural foods; women's clothing; skincare products; fitness books, CDs, and tapes; healing products; tours, retreats, workshops, and conferences; and teacher training and educational programming. The remaining substantive pieces are dedicated to how-to, self-care articles helpful to teachers and students; advice for managing one's life; informative pieces about yoga and its notable teachers; and practice opportunities. Issues beyond the physicality of asana practice (e.g., working with desires or focusing one's awareness) are handled in twenty pages. Most material is geared toward fitness- and health-oriented aspects of practice.

And who are *Yoga Journal's* targeted consumers? Women, of course. More than three-fourths of some three hundred images of models and others are females, typically under forty. This roughly approximates the average gender distribution in many yoga classes across the country today. In fact, almost all of the magazine's cover models from April 2002 to April 2008 were young, attractive women. When the few cover men appeared, they were restricted to renowned middle-aged teachers like Rod Stryker, John Friend, or Richard Freeman. Given the trends and advertising that feed yoga's growth, it is not surprising that a national online survey of practitioners finds the average yoga student to be a female in her mid-thirties, also a perfect target market for readers.[24]

## The Business of Yoga

The development of a yoga industry is in the very nature of American cultural life and its incestuous intertwining with business. Anything that can be melted down into a product line or service that is exotic, unique, beneficial, and saleable to any age group, race, or creed is certain to be borrowed, replicated, imitated, and packaged for profit. Yoga is only the latest in the line of products and services—pizza, coffeehouses, and football among them—that are creatively altered, franchised, and even re-exported for sale back to their points of origin.

Once reduced to asana, yoga's most recent product differentiation now takes the form of laughter yoga, yogilates (yoga and pilates), yoga spin (yoga and cycling), and yo-chi (yoga and t'ai chi).[25] In Los Angeles—capital of creative chaos—yoga's ancient ecology has been thrown off balance as it has been hybridized to include ballet yoga, kick-box yoga, and hip-hop yoga. "They appear to be reinventing yoga by drawing inspiration from other physical training systems," says Ramaswami, while "some of the basic tenets, like slow breathing and mind focus, are being put aside."[26] More careful grafting occurs at weekend retreat programs, where traditional yoga practice is combined with golf, knitting, tango, and creative writing. The appearance of franchised and chain studios with creative options for doing asanas was only a question of time, especially since the health care and fitness industries had already gone down that commercial road. America's ubiquitous chain stores had also entered the lucrative sales market for yoga gear.

Yoga's transformation may be epitomized by the all-inclusive yoga vacation plan. Advertisements beckon the practitioner with magazine photos of yoginis in triangle pose on mountaintops and sunny tropical beaches, as magazine articles tout upscale yoga vacations. This should not surprise anyone. After all, Americanization means that the packaging of this holistic lifestyle into a leisure pursuit is only natural in a society wedded to ceaseless work and busyness and our resulting need for rest and relaxation once freed from job responsibilities. What could fit this need better than yoga, now placed in the same category as running, hiking, and biking as fun activities?

Yet business packaging means more than providing entertainment outlets for yoga lovers. Conferences offer hundreds of human potential workshops around the country each year and advertise through catalogs, target mailers, Web sites, and magazines, including *Yoga Journal.* They also accommodate our work and leisure lives with three- to seven-day intensives ranging from the silly and sublime to the sacred and significant. Positive feeling, palpable lightness, and open exploration permeate these offerings directed at a decidedly middle-class and professional clientele. More serious practitioners pick and choose to match their personal interests among America's top teachers, psychotherapists, scientists, specialty practitioners, and indigenous healers. At the same time, yoga business-packaging is being actively globalized. The 2007 Asia Yoga Conference gave top billing to America's celebrity teachers while honoring one of its great patriarchs, K. Patabhi Jois, who had fostered yoga's growth on U.S. soil by training many of its teachers in India over the past four decades.

A crucial question curdling to the top of this business brew is how yoga's integrity as a spiritual practice can be effectively maintained as it becomes just another entrée in the glut of products and services awaiting their turn as grist in the commercial mill of postmodern life. With some sense of alarm at these developments, Cushman pondered on the pages of her magazine: "In a country—and an era—when consumerism is itself a kind of religion, spiritual marketing seems to have reached new heights of glossy sophistication. The superficiality is no less rampant in the world of Hatha yoga, where spiritual enlightenment is often measured by how good you look in a leotard." For Cushman, the challenge before the burgeoning yoga industry was to find "a way of letting inspiration flow through us, without believing that it's our inspiration."[27]

Cushman captures yoga's uniquely contemporary bipolar condition—a business enterprise and spiritual path packaged into creative fitness workouts and specialized workshops. Yoga's bipolarity appears to pose a serious danger to the health of a noble ancient path and may warrant some metaphorical medication as a corrective. The challenge for leaders of this fee-for-service growth industry—its magazine editors, book writers, renowned teachers, and retreat directors—is how they will respond to these developments that so vitally affect yoga's future. Will they press their energies to "buck the trend," or will they reconcile with or actively promote more of the fitness flow of yoga dough? Many retreat center presidents, studio owners, and teachers around the country recognize the need to strike a balance—if not to address the tension between—the requirements of traditional yoga spirituality and the business demands of a far more lucrative marketplace. Their decisions reflect their perspectives and priorities and those of their organizations, and ultimately will affect that of the public as well.

CHAPTER 3 THREE

# Filling the Big Tent

The yoga world has expanded to become big business—a mainstream health and fitness phenomenon. A case in point is the three-day yoga conference and trade show in Toronto in May 2006. In advance of the extravaganza, promotional materials touted twenty-five thousand attendees, 125 workshops, cross-training classes on yoga for athletes, live entertainment, and 250 exhibitors selling everything from alternative medicine to Zen home décor. The extravaganza itself featured long lines at check-in, substantial registration fees, large hotel ballrooms covered with yoga mats, sales of commercial accessories—books, clothing, DVDs, videos, natural oils, scents, vacations, and retreats—and other characteristics of a hot marketplace.

Yoga Group, Inc. claims that between 2003 and 2005 there was a 41 percent increase in yoga practitioners in the United States, according to a nationwide survey. *Yoga Journal*'s paid circulation tripled between 1998 and 2005, and at least two-thirds of health-and-fitness facilities now offer yoga, with its proportion doubling in six years.[1] That is a major shift from thirty years ago, when yoga practitioners viewed spirituality as more central to the practice, regarded a physical workout as a side benefit of yoga, and hardly considered yoga's potential as a mass-market enterprise.

Does yoga's foray into the world of commerce automatically mean it must lose its deep roots? Can a healthy balance exist between yoga's spiritual and material sides? There are no easy answers to these questions, as yoga-centered businesses sensitive to these issues struggle to find a middle ground.

## Inner History, Outer Change

The Kripalu Center for Yoga and Health near Lenox, Massachusetts, clearly reveals the evolving face of yoga. As a spiritual retreat and education center challenged to run as a profit-oriented business, Kripalu must thrive and expand by offering what its current customers want. Yet its teachings continue to adhere to its mission and to provide educational experiences in transformative consciousness. Can the Center find the balance to incorporate all aspects of yoga into one big tent, and can it strengthen its roots without watering them down? My interviews with key people, as I relay below, help address these questions.

Kripalu president Garrett Sarley, known as Dinabhandu, puts the issue this way:

> The American approach to yoga has a downside, in that it has become more materialistic, more 'body only,' more shallow. The upside is that if twenty million are practicing it, that is all to the good. You get this cross-training, this openness, this effervescence and creativity. It comes down to how you keep skillful in the depth and breadth as well as the creativity of yoga.

There lies the opportunity and the threat. And Kripalu just might be up to the challenge of creating and maintaining the balancing act. It is a place where mysticism meets pragmatism, along with wisdom, compassion, experiential learning, warm smiles, and easy laughter.

An hour's drive from Albany International Airport, a winding, wooded road leads to a five-acre red brick building overlooking Lake Mahkeenac in the Berkshire Mountains of western Massachusetts. This is a road well-traveled, out of sheer love for the place, on my eight trips in five years. Called Shadowbrook, the building and adjacent land were once owned by wealthy industrialist Andrew Carnegie. The Jesuit order later occupied the property for two decades. Kripalu moved to this site in 1981, about a decade after its founding as an ashram in rural Pennsylvania. Inside the building, framed sayings of Mother Theresa, the Dalai Lama, Mohandas Gandhi, and Dr. Martin Luther King Jr. decorate stairwell walls.

Kripalu spirituality is a juicy, paradoxical potage with spicy Indian philosophical influences. It includes Vedantic nondualism, where God and Soul are One; devotional and selfless service; Hatha yoga and its stepparent *Tantra;* and *The Yoga Sutra*'s spirit-nature dualism. These influences are mixed in with dedication to Shiva, the phallic god of transformation, and Ganapati, the beloved elephant-headed deity whose statue greets travelers at the back entrance. Spiritual seekers and senior practitioners once embodied Swami Kripalu's kundalini yogic ideal and that of his charismatic student and heir Amrit Desai. The overarching Indian worldview offered a blueprint for enlightenment that embodied ethical precepts, dietary requirements, daily yoga and meditation, and mantra practice, including kirtan, or melodious devotional chanting. Kripalu was primarily a haven for those committed to transformation.

After a sex scandal rocked the ashram in 1994, the community underwent dramatic and wrenching change. Desai was asked to leave, and Kripalu faced the legal and financial repercussions of organizational restructuring. By the late 1990s, Kripalu had recast itself as a "meta-university"—an educational center dedicated to personal, societal, and global transformation—replete with a reconstituted board, new bylaws, paid employees, and an expanding range of holistic health services for clients and trainees alike. While these changes may have meant stepping out from the traditional paradigm, they were also a giant step toward embracing the outside world.

At about the same time, yoga as asana practice began to grow in popularity throughout the country. As we have seen, magazines, talk shows, movies, and Internet sites promoted celebrity practitioners, and yoga's substantial health benefits were touted to a public riding an economic boom. It did not take long for the larger expendable incomes to be invested at Kripalu for classes and retreats of various types, stylized mats and props, books and clothing, scents and music, and teas and food.

## Transforming Space

As the shift took place at Kripalu, one of the Center's challenges was to skillfully address the full-scale secularization of yoga. Would it be a threat or an opportunity for the organization, or both? Would Kripalu's strengths be cultivated or weaknesses exposed as it addressed this cultural and economic change? What balance could be forged, what transformation undertaken?

Confronting serious fiscal challenges, Kripalu hired Dinabhandu as president in 2004 and gave him an active role on the Board of Trustees. A past president of the Omega Institute, a large New Age retreat center in New York, Dinabhandu had been a resident monk at Kripalu in the 1970s. If anyone could walk the new yogic balance beam, it seemed he would be the one. Essentially, Dinabhandu was hired to address the organizational challenges of maintaining a space committed to transformation in a changing environment. Kripalu's resident scholar Stephen Cope has written that "the best transformational space must always be preparing the ground for its own transformation."[2] The Kripalu Center seemed to embody that principle under new leadership.

"It's quite radical, what we're trying to do," remarked Dinabhandu about his vision for Kripalu as a meta-university:

> We're trying to articulate, or bring into being, an entirely new kind of institution. If you say, 'I want higher education,' people will say, 'Go to a college or university.' If you say, 'I want to involve myself in music,' they will say, 'Check out a conservatory or symphony.' Those are common responses in society. But if you say, 'I want to be more myself, be more fulfilled and powerful in my being,' it would be unclear where you could go.

Kripalu's leadership, including Dinabhandu's new management team, actualized Dinabhandu's vision by planning for expansion of Shadowbrook—diversifying its housing, program rooms, and public spaces; adding an integrated healing center and new landscaping; and expanding the donor base. Programs reportedly increased from five hundred to nine hundred in the first year under his leadership, with greater accessibility for more individuals. Twenty-five thousand visited Shadowbrook in 2006 alone.

The current approach guiding Kripalu is not based on a traditional business model, at least not at its core. "I did a long report to the board outlining the strategy and tactics, mission and principles," Dinabhandu told me. "In the end, I understand the need for that. But because we're not trying to be someplace in five years, that's not the discipline we are leading from." He uses the analogy of yoga practice:

> It is similar to a posture. You can say that I would like to have my forehead on my knees in the forward bend. But then you start to do it; to get there, you might injure yourself. So your discipline is not putting your head to your knees; it is embodying yoga in your particular body at that particular time with that particular flexibility in that particular posture.

> So asking, 'What is your strategic plan?' is like asking in yoga class, 'Where do you want to be in five years?' It's so important to lead in a gradual, open way rather than in a corporate way.

Regardless of the vision and strategy, difficult organizational changes are necessary. Dinabhandu notes: "High-performing teams have more life-force energy than low-performing teams. So we have very high standards of performance, and if you don't meet them, you lose your job."

## Views from the Center

Robin Lamperti spent more than sixty days at Kripalu between 2004 and 2006, working toward a five hundred-hour yoga teacher certification. A partner in an information security consulting business before opening her Neponset Valley Yoga Studio outside of Boston, Lamperti has seen the transformation at Kripalu firsthand and in a very short time. "There are a lot of changes happening at Kripalu now," she said to me. "A lot of the people who I consider embodying Kripalu yoga will be moving on. I want to learn from these people before they are gone."

Lamperti experienced changes in guest attitudes, personnel shuffles, and dietary expansion. The professional and ancillary staff is especially sensitive to these changes. Some have decided to leave because of them; others have been asked to leave. Bittersweet is the result—some anger and sadness met by opportunity and openness to change. "When it was a spiritual center, it attracted a certain type of person, a spiritual seeker," Lamperti says. "Now that they have transitioned from being a spiritual center, they are attracting more of the mainstream population. They are doing what they need to do to stay financially viable. But with meat on the menu, what about *ahimsa* [nonaggression]?"

Despite concerns about shifting from a vegetarian menu to one that includes chicken and fish, Lamperti is positive about the changes:

> Kripalu has always been evolving, ever since it was born in this country. So in many ways, I am excited for them about the change. Having run a successful company, I understand that economics drive your business, whether you want it to or not. It is a tricky thing to balance integrity and heart with financial liability. So if Kripalu continues to deliver programs with heart, I think they will be fine. . . . They are beginning to attract a lot of big names, which is attracting more people.

Indeed, a cursory look at Kripalu's year-round offerings reads like a "Who's Who" of American yoga—Rodney Yee, Ana Forrest, Shiva Rea, Rod Stryker, Cyndi Lee, and a host of second-tier teachers. "Their ability to put together programs amazes me. The way they bring something to production is phenomenal," says Lamperti. The extensive programming encourages students to return, allows its reputation to grow, and provides the financial means to move forward. By 2006, Kripalu had added a Sacred Pulse Music Festival of dancing, drumming, and chanting with nationally known kirtan masters, as well as the Ashtanga Mela Gathering—an "ultimate yoga vacation" with renowned teachers, music, stories, and feasts. The not-for-profit also started up a transformational leadership program for eighteen- to twenty-five-year-olds as well as a comprehensive yoga research program to add "rigor and integrity" to the ancient practice.

And what will this shift toward diversification and inclusion of the mainstream portend for Kripalu's own style of yoga?

## Learning to Swim

Besides expanding winning programs, another growth strategy of the Center is to deliberately separate Kripalu yoga from Kripalu as a retreat organization. Kripalu yoga offers a contemplative approach to the discipline, leading from the willful and deliberate action of beginning practice to the surrendering of will and effort and the spontaneous play and sacred dance of advanced practice known as *sahaja* yoga. Lamperti notes:

> As an organization, it is a facility and retreat center and needs to be sustainable. They want to find out if Kripalu yoga is viable by letting it out in the deep end of the pool to see if it can swim. It has been supported by the organization for a lot of years. All the teachers and trainings have been proprietary to the building. As teachers go on the road, they will see if Kripalu yoga can survive outside the building in Lenox.

At the same time, teacher-training sessions for other yoga styles have been slotted for Shadowbrook, including a popular program headed by Rodney Yee.

Michael Carroll, also known as Yoganand, is a senior member of Kripalu and past director of the yoga teacher-training program. He owns his own studio, Radiant Well-Being Yoga, in North Augusta, South Carolina. As he explains it, yoga teacher training has been lucrative for the Kripalu organization, and nothing is likely to change that. "Recently we had over seventy trainees for a YTT [Yoga Teacher Training] program, the largest group since the early nineties," which was *before* the yoga boom and proliferation of training programs nationwide. He is grateful that he can continue to lead teacher-training programs off-site, where he is free to improvise with the format and bring greater rigor as well as launch his own accredited training program.

Today, Kripalu the organization is a business enterprise with a menu of products and services that is riding the yoga wave to become one of America's major yoga resources. Yoganand and other teachers who operate as fee-for-service employees are old friends who form their own communities at Kripalu. Newer members such as

Lamperti do the same, finding a spiritual subculture within this more bottom-line driven organization.

With such flexibility in mind, Kripalu seems to be broadening its original purpose by promoting yoga as a revitalizing agent for society and as a resource for those with different stylistic tastes and motivations. "Standing for integrative consciousness, we're not trying to fight one or the other—spiritual or material yoga—but to 'up-level' everything," explains Dinabhandu. "If you want to de-stress in your job, we can teach you to do that, and if we do, we think the chance of your going deeper is greater. But if that is all you want to learn, that's fine too."

Originally, Kripalu was the vision of a renunciate not particularly interested in the material world. "Yoga here has always been from the inside out. That's always been its strength," asserts Dinabhandu. "But we have tried to bring awareness of other schools of yoga. We are trying to have the institution be a big tent. Different approaches to yoga are appropriate for different types of people and different phases in life." Perhaps Kripalu's newly evolving mantra is merely responding to consumer need. Is it also surrendering its original vision? The answer lies with one's perspective toward an evolving yoga and its differentiated subculture.

## The Bigger Picture

Kripalu's changes will inevitably have an effect on what people think of the organization as well as its yoga style. As a studio owner, Lamperti also walks this balance, running a yoga business committed to being profitable yet teaching practices inherent in Kripalu yoga as a lifestyle path. She offers a warning for any future tampering in which Kripalu loses its essence: "People who have done Kripalu yoga like it. But there are so many styles, and people want to try all of them. Yet from a pure marketing standpoint, it is easier for me to offer something that is clearly branded."

With growing commercialism come not only organizational challenges but the possibility of initiating real change in how people ultimately view and treat themselves. More yoga options will mean little if the art of living—yoga's wisdom center—is not used as a beacon for bringing about change in the personal lives of its practitioners. Kripalu's greatest challenge—and the challenge of thousands of other "yoga businesses"—lies less with transforming its organization or expanding its style of yoga. These businesses may best serve by providing the millions of yoga newcomers with opportunities for redemption from any punitive or overly ambitious outlook. Managing such inner transformation, from "body as machine" to "body as receptacle of sacred life-force energy," is an integral part of yogic teaching and learning.

Referring to newcomers' secular and overly physical outlook, Lamperti says, "It is almost as if some people feel they need to be punished somehow—through a punishing workout. The way some religion is practiced in this country, if there is an element of sin or punishment or shame in it, people are attracted to it. It also translates into the type of yoga they are attracted to." She adds, "People are attracted to things that test them in ways that are not necessarily spiritually supportive; rather, they feel that this is what they 'deserve.'" Yoga as a punitive practice contrasts sharply with the traditional approach embodied in the classic Indian school of Hatha yoga, where postures should be comfortable and not painful, naturally freeing muscles and skeletal connections.

Commercial extravaganzas like the Yoga in Toronto Conference and Show guarantee continuous performances, demonstrations, and lectures that yoga consumers have come to expect at major events. Profits easily follow, along with growing public accessibility and interest. While providing a forum for practitioners to celebrate their community, these extravaganzas give lip service to yoga's roots. At free seminars and demonstrations, Toronto attendees had the opportunity to learn how to apply the path more fully to their lives, with a chance to experience a nonintimidating glimpse of yoga as something beyond the typical hour-and-a-half workout. But this is only a first step in this ancient practice's promise of personal transformation, in a society where practicing poses is what most students want and what the general public associates with the term "yoga."

While a more superficial, commercial side of the practice is challenged to contain a spiritual message, traditional retreat centers have a similar charge to maintain their integrity within the expanded space required by yoga's enormous popularity. The real sin and shame would be to leave the impression that this sacred dance, this energetic celebration should be bought and sold, stripped down, and rebranded in ways that disrespect its transformative value as a holistic way of life. Venerable ashrams and resourceful retreat centers have an ethical and societal responsibility to protect themselves as containers for deeper practice, especially if all that many consumers want is fitness, fun, physical challenge, and material comfort. Kripalu Center has charted its course. Only time will tell if the Center continues to offer America what it always had—the "real deal" of yoga spirituality.

CHAPTER FOUR

# Making It on Broadway

On a hot and sultry afternoon, I entered Namaste Yoga and Healing Center on Broadway in downtown Asheville, North Carolina and asked the tall, slender man with beard and dreadlocks if he owned the place. "Well, of course, the Lord is really in charge. But yes, I run this center," he said. His name is Sean, and like many other owners of spiritual yoga centers, his Namaste has attracted a community coalescing around its yoga classes, programs, and retreats. For some locals, Asheville's valley home is considered a natural healing ground, as it was for native people long ago, and the center extends its ancient function to a progressive urban community.

Like other centers currently dotting the country, this one attracts freethinkers who form a distinct culture of transformative consciousness—what was more commonly called "New Age culture" a decade or two ago. Through the center's offerings—Hatha yoga, chanting, workshops, vegan meals, incense, and related products—a local community defines itself in this hip, artsy nook of the Southeast. It all looks and feels healthy and balanced on the surface, but how does it sustain yoga as a transformative path?

Serious students of any authentic practice know that theirs is a challenging yet beneficial one. It depends on continued diligence, determination, and love while offering no money-back guarantee. With time, patience, and practice, students feel more resilient and open, more loving and compassionate. To be properly represented, an authentic practice cannot be packaged as a quick fix for consumers accustomed to thinking in terms of finding instant solutions for physical challenges, psychological issues, or spiritual malaise. Balancing authenticity with consumer expectations is the challenge for centers committed to yoga's foundational principles in light of New Age culture's transformation into a business market segment.

## Mainstreaming the Alternative

As yoga is being transformed frontally by commercial interests that shrink it down to a fitness regimen, its flank is exposed by association with the changing character of the New Age. This cultural phenomenon has been a peculiar incubator for yoga in America, keeping it alive in the 1980s as a viable discipline with deep philosophical roots while linking it in the minds of some Americans with edgy, offbeat, and at times thoroughly nutty ideas. In one sense, New Age culture has been yoga's cute, sweet, smiling stepsister, donning a colorful peasant dress while seated barefoot on the porch—promoting an airy spirituality of chanting sessions, paraphernalia for practice, *puja* purifications, and a circuit of traveling teachers. In another way, New Age culture has been yoga's psychotic stepmother channeling a fifty-thousand-year-old being for the more gullible while balancing a healing pyramid on her head down in the basement.

Whereas yoga is a serious pathway for personal metamorphosis, its ambivalent relationship with New Age culture may profit from some serious evaluation. Looking under the surface at yoga centers like Namaste in Asheville drives the point home: Services offered to those with New Age sensibilities must be carefully balanced with the integrity of yoga spirituality.

The New Age is only the most recent of romantic subcultures that have resided on the fringe of Western society. Others have gained respectability or disappeared to a trash heap of interesting historical idiosyncrasies. Holistic health theories and practices once considered "alternative" have initiated positive changes in the health care industry over the past thirty years. Yoga, massage, reiki, reflexology, meditation, indigenous healing, and other forms of therapeutic work are successful as niche, more mainstream, and complementary health practices.

Assimilation of the New Age's more intellectual side—theories on the borderline of conventional science and spirituality—has not been as easy. Yet Ken Wilber, Charles Tart, Stanislav Grof, Theodore Roszak, Rupert Sheldrake, and Fritjof Capra are the well-respected senior citizenry of the 1980s-style consciousness revolution. They represent the New Age's concern for the interconnection between person and planet and hint at yoga's role in the process. The stereotyped flakiness of what was thought of as New Age—crystal healing, wheat germ and yeast cures, aura sprays, Christ's hidden years, and extraterrestrial angels—has by and large faded from the public's mind while esoteric traditions, yoga, and sustainable technology have captured the attention of popular media and advertising alike.

*Natural* is the operative word underlying the New Age's real success story and its sustaining cultural legacy—preserving what is healthy in being human and finding expression in natural foods, fibers, festivals, feelings, healings, and energies. All these, as its adherents explain, are necessary healing products, services, and experiences for the stresses of living in our complex, consumer-driven society. Since we need to be made whole again, the New Age has furnished answers for personal and planetary health. One answer is to borrow and synthesize practices of native peoples from around the world, those who live closer to the natural and energetic rhythms of life—be it through Celtic pagan celebrations, Native

American sweat lodges, Asian spiritual traditions, or World music. Another answer has been to create new systems for renewal, taking ancient notions while grafting on contemporary-sounding ideas.

Consider some labels so easily associated today with those committed to personal or planetary health and to what is natural: Pagans, Greens, vegetarians, fiber artists, yogis, massage therapists, and solar-heating devotees. Add to them the countless millions predisposed to herbs, botanicals, meditation, massage, wilderness preservation, and alternate fuel sources. With slow assimilation of holistic health practices and the ramping up of the economy through the 1990s, those committed to living healthy lifestyles with an ecological consciousness could afford to invest more money in support of their personal commitments. Positively portrayed, this creative class and their lifestyle converts have become an evolving market segment with an air of respectability for business. While many may not identify with the term "New Age" at all, they share similar tastes in music, literature, symbols, language, politics, health care, art, entertainment, business acumen, and spirituality.

Those dedicated to personal and planetary health espouse what marketers refer to as "LOHAS:" Lifestyles of Health and Sustainability.[1] They comprise an estimated seventeen percent of adults who buy eco-friendly products of all kinds; read self-help, spiritual, and psychotherapy books; are attracted to yoga and meditation; and understand their lives through the prism of spiritual (as opposed to religious) worldviews. Ariana Speyer of Beliefnet.com defines these Americans as "metrospirituals"—those who have the discretionary income and personal commitment to purchase based on their holistic values and who are mainstreaming Eastern religions like Hinduism and Buddhism into "an easily-digestible, buyable form."[2] The metrospiritual phenomenon is very good news for the business side of yoga and a potential challenge for those committed to authentic spiritual practice.

## The Business of Spiritual Yoga

Sean Bookman, the thirty-three-year-old owner of Namaste, "moved to consciousness" and to Asheville to set up shop six years ago. Namaste is one of many multifaceted centers dedicated to holistic yoga and to the healing arts. Traditional Indian technologies for transformation are offered in the form of retreats and workshops to those interested and willing to pay. Centers like Namaste provide welcome benefits to their local LOHAS communities, which are the basis for their material success.

After garnering a six-figure income in the travel sales and advertising industry, Sean and wife Nicole decided to focus their lives on what was most important to them—their spiritual development. He's a Rastafarian from New Jersey with strong marketing and sales skills; she is a mother and yoga teacher with a visionary seed that bore fruit.

Nicole was raised in Texas and met Sean at the Los Angeles House of Blues, where she worked for founder Isaac Tigrett, a disciple of renowned Indian master Sai Baba. "There are pictures and quotes of Sai Baba everywhere, and you have the option to take yoga, which he makes available to his staff. All of that began to intrigue me," she said. Nicole also attended classes during a short stay in northern California, and when Sean took a job in Miami, she found her passion: "I loved what I learned in yoga. I knew this was my path, and I found what I was going to do with the rest of my life." Completing her two hundred-hour teacher training with Prana Yoga, she moved with Sean to Asheville with the intention of opening a yoga center in its downtown of quaint shops and restaurants.

As its Web site proclaims, Sean and Nicole's yoga center was established "for those who seek the true essence in themselves and wish to be in a like-minded community. From the moment you walk into the center, your stresses are melted away. The Zen and spa-like environment helps bring you back into balance." Here, it is easy to ground oneself in more meditative asana practice as its teachers cover many Yogic traditions—Ananda, Ashtanga, Kripalu, Sivananada, and Kundalini.

"It's a bit of a balancing act for us," Sean admits. "Even though it's a spiritual center, a community center, it's still a business." The current economics of the yoga business mean that owners must find ways to keep their mission clear while giving students what they want. "We hardly make money at all on yoga classes," says Nicole. "We charge thirteen dollars, and the teacher gets half of that. What keeps us open is the special events and retreats, retail, and the food. To tell you the truth, if we brought in pilates or hot yoga, we would pack the place. But that is not who we are; it is not our path, our niche." With a strong interest in family-centered yoga, she teaches prenatal yoga, postnatal yoga with baby, toddler yoga, and children's yoga. They are among Namaste's biggest class revenue generators.

The Bookmans have created a center for transformation and healing in an area that naturally attracts teachers and seekers from around the world. Some parts of the country are magnets for those committed to a higher consciousness associated with LOHAS—healing and arts communities like Sedona, Taos, and Asheville; university towns like Ithaca, Boulder, Austin, and Madison; and progressive and youthful cities like Seattle and Portland. Collectively, they happen to be the bluest of American locales—hotbeds of liberalism, progressive third-party and anti-war politics, and ecological sensitivity.

As Sean puts it, "Asheville is protected by these ancient mountains, and it has long been known as a healing valley. When I first came here on business, I felt something very strong." Yoga, meditation, and other sources of healing are the vehicles for serving its inhabitants while creating a profitable business. In Asheville, Sean and Nicole began to attract a bevy of the area's many seekers as well as renowned teachers and healers from Asia, Africa, and Latin America who regularly rotate through their Blue Ridge Mountain community.

Tibetan monk Geshe Michael Roach once visited their community. "I could see his white aura emanate as he was talking about taking away suffering from other people," Sean recalls. Another time, Bhagavan Das and Wah! performed their powerful kirtans: "All of a sudden everyone was smiling, standing, dancing, and chanting, 'Jai ma.' Everyone could feel it; they were so bright and leaving the center full of love." Shakta Kaur Khalsa also visited, and Hare Krishnas rented space at Namaste. A large chanting community grew weekly, and classes filled the available time slots.

The magnetism of the space and the magic of the place meant that Namaste would more than make it: "Feeling that divine connection and spreading it around, a reputation for authentic spiritual experience" is how Sean explains why the center has grown. Now the job is to keep to what is pure and clear—no power yoga or purely fitness forms—and to separate the deeper wheat from the less authentic chaff—turning away programs by those noted more for tantric sex than for Tantric yoga.

Nicole says that it is a challenge to remain profitable:

> Unfortunately, to get some teachers, it costs an outrageous amount, at a minimum. That's the balance right there—trying to keep Namaste a place where people can afford to come and yet meet our profit margin. Then there are a lot of people who don't feel they should have to pay for spiritual knowledge at all. But it takes money to keep a center open, to keep things alive. We are still 'month-to-month.' It's a tight budget. If you want to be super-rich, this is not the business to be in unless you go super-corporate and franchise.

And many others have.

## Offerings and Outcomes

Sean and Nicole's contribution to their wider community—like that of LOHAS culture's to America at large—lies in the various ways that Namaste addresses the human need for meaningful transformation. Nicole says, "We are just a humble little family trying to be of service to ourselves, to the community, to God, to a higher good for humanity, making a better world for our children and our children's children."

Workshops are offered year-round and are important moneymakers in sustaining the center. In the spirit of the New Age, Namaste's cleansing retreats for the wider community provide detoxification through asanas, *kriyas*, massage, meditation, pranayama, kirtan, herbal cleansing, organic meals, and communal purifications. The search here is for finding natural balance, which resonates well with the Yogic worldview. "Namaste offers opportunities through workshops and programs for that individual spark to be struck," Nicole says.

> There are no promises of outcome. Yoga is an individual journey. All we can do is facilitate a place where they can come and put them in an environment that will encourage the inner growth that is inside them. Sometimes there is internal resistance, and you just hope that with time they will continue to come and find that quiet space inside themselves. You can have two people with the same teacher, and one can reach samadhi and the other will not.

Yet the challenge for any business in an environment brimming with opportunity is to ensure that its portrayal of products or services is consistent with what it eventually provides. For centers of transformative yoga, this potential tension between the business side—offering beneficial services—and the spiritual side—where there is no money-back guarantee—is all the more palatable.

Namaste contributes to the recovery of a healing balance by providing practitioners the means for reconnecting with themselves and their earth through its offerings. While it must advertise to stay in business, can it be inviting without the benefits of participation sounding too airy, easy, or assuring? Can Namaste and other like organizations fulfill their mission without having to hype benefits at all?

Consider these advertised promises of workshops and retreats nationwide. The Namaste Web site describes one of its healing retreats this way:

> *Japa*, or repetition of the Divine Name, is the most important of all yogic practices and the easiest path to realizing our true self. Next, we will explore the breath and its relation to our mind through the exercise of breath restraint. Through the control of prana (life force) we can now ride the Divine Name home in perfect unbroken remembrance of our true self and fall into meditation of *Dhyana*, by the Divine grace.

Another organization's retreat in Arizona promises that

> we can bring you into harmony with the voices of the land and sky. . . . The stark beauty and raw power of Nature will inspire the communion you've been longing for. We can show you how to access the wisdom of your own body and soul. Master teachers and healers will lead you to the heart of your life. You will feel your own power. You will hear the voice of your own soul. You will experience the love of God directly. . . . You will discover why you were born.

A twelve-day Caribbean retreat set up by a Florida firm suggests that dolphins, as "conscious breathers," must

> remain awake in order to breathe. In other words, they 'remain in the present' (as yogis of the seas!), and perhaps it is this state of conscious awareness that humans find so magical and magnetic. We like to take this lesson from the dolphins and work with the breath, using yoga and other techniques such as the Quantum Light breath meditation. . . . [Participants will find that] the combination of yoga, healthy food, cruising, and relaxing on the boat on the clear, warm aquamarine ocean and being with the dolphins adds to our spiritual health and healing.

A workshop featuring a nationally known teacher of kundalini yoga is advertised as follows: "Find out about the Kundalini energy and how it is awakened with Kundalini Yoga, the 'mother yoga.' . . . Have a complete Kundalini Yoga experience, which includes powerfully elevating yoga, deep relaxation, and divine music and meditation in the Kundalini tradition."

While the language fits the needs and interests of many on the metrospiritual market, a skeptic might question if these offerings can deliver the real deal. Do these marketable descriptions, or can any pitch, do justice to balancing business needs with spiritual mission? As with all advertising, the devil is in the details, and with services promoting transformative consciousness, it is critical neither to oversell nor to under-promise. After all, *complete* kundalini experiences are truly difficult to accomplish even for the most serious of yogis who practice for a lifetime, since these experiences demand a one-pointed, wholehearted commitment to practice while holding no guarantees of a positive outcome. Yet some practitioners *do* have glimpses or experiences of the ultimate nature of things—in the *turiya* state of deep meditative awareness beyond waking, dreaming, and sleeping where the blissful witness consciousness naturally dawns.

Great masters are said to live their entire lives in that state. One of them was Lama Yeshe, the late Tibetan teacher of Tantra yoga.

He had found that "many Westerners are extremely impatient; they want instant results. They buy instant coffee, instant soup, instant breakfast, instant everything. And when it comes to the spiritual path they want instant satisfaction, instant experiences."[3]

Are business and spiritual intentions mutually contradictory? Some teachers from the East have actively marketed the benefits of the practices they teach. Yet authentic yogic spirituality asks us to practice over the long term, with awareness of yoga's benefits, with an intense desire to overcome our suffering but without attachment to the specific outcome (i.e., freedom or release). However, business advertising is directly interested in promising tangible and often easily attainable benefits to its consumers as a motivation to seal the deal. This tension between spirituality and business advertising appears to be the central challenge for any center offering a deeper, more holistic approach to yoga in America today.

## Seeking Sobriety

Centers that prioritize yoga spirituality offer opportunities through workshops and programs for a transformative spark to be struck in those sympathetic to LOHAS sensitivities. Yet advertising any promise of outcome may make it seem too simple to accomplish a higher and more blissful awareness. That is the problem: Advertising of any kind is by its very nature part truth and part propaganda, often written to the lowest common denominator while geared toward those lacking the time, patience, or knowledge to study the fine print. In tradition-based yoga, that fine print has always read as follows: "Commitment to years of practice is required. Do so with the goal in mind but without concern for the outcome. Having a spiritually gifted teacher is highly recommended." Perhaps the many yoga centers in this country that make a difference in so many people's lives need to place that warning label in boldface.

Yet linking practice to claims of benefit makes such logical sense. After all, practices like yoga have a menu of benefits that manifest among practitioners and that are essentially true: Yoga can reduce stress and tension. It can act as an antidepressant. It will activate the lymphatic system to prevent disease. It does empower the heart to lead us to a more profound love. Yoga can and does produce all of these results, but (and this is the point) it does so only for those serious enough to dedicate themselves to the path over the long term and perhaps not solely through the workshop road to fitness, rehabilitation, or enlightenment. It is small wonder that officials at the National Institutes for Health (NIH) in Bethesda, Maryland were initially reluctant to take up studies of yoga and other healing practices, lest the research be tainted by association with what can sound at times like "crackpot medicine" with wild, unmeasured, or unsubstantiated claims.

Many well-intentioned people are committed to bringing about positive, meaningful change for themselves and their communities. Millions "live LOHAS" and make a wonderful difference in a world with its litany of problems. However, promoting a practice by dangling psychophysical-spiritual outcomes in front of buyers on the marketplace may lead to a misunderstanding of yoga spirituality that matches the workout industry's fitness misinterpretation.

A sober assessment of the business side of America's LOHAS culture may be needed, especially if the integrity of yoga as a holistic discipline is to be strengthened. This assessment has much less to do with critiquing the values that underlie the culture's basic intention—helping us to become more fully human in a more harmonious world—or with criticizing the many gifted Seans and loving Nicoles who are committed to making America truly spirit-centered. Rather, the assessment should ask how opportunities for transformation are portrayed through services for sale.

A constant challenge for spiritual yoga centers is giving primacy to deeper transformation in its balancing act with business. As Nicole has put it,

> We do have projected business plans for Namaste. But it's about keeping true and expanding. There is a fine line there. You have to assure that the authentic vibration remains with it. Namaste has kind of developed by itself. We really don't own it; we facilitate it. It has grown into its own identity, and we are just grateful to all the people who come and support it. It all comes back to our own path, where we are growing and how it can all work together.

So added to the profit-oriented fitness centers that are transforming American yoga by feeding its popularity is an uneasy integration of LOHAS's spiritual yoga with business acumen. Given the commercial forces currently at play, maintaining the integrity of yoga as a deeper discipline requires a reassessment of its current relationship to business or to any source touting either easy accomplishment or unrealizable expectation. This means bringing metrospirituality out of the New Age cellar, off its business porch, and up onto its lofty rooftop where the air is clearer, the music lighter, and one's footing is more secure for practicing yoga's traditions while suspending concern for either benefit or outcome.

CHAPTER 5 FIVE

# Temple and Club

"*Om Namah Shivaya . . . Om Namo Bhagavate . . . Hara Hara MahaDeva . . .* " These sacred mantras, timeless sounds of classical Indian chants fused with a mild percussion beat, may be in the background while practitioners do yoga poses, sit in meditation, or do the dishes. They can transform us, relax and open us, or even entertain us. Around the world, kirtan music is filling ashrams, retreat centers, temples, yoga studios, rented facilities, homes, and anywhere people gather to celebrate and acknowledge their love of life with joyful chants. Traditionally, kirtan is ancient melodious chanting that calls upon primordial energy in the form of gods and goddesses of the Hindu pantheon. The mantras invoke these psycho-spiritual energies as expressions of our true nature, for both deeper and mundane ends. They are central to the Bhakti and Tantric paths to spiritual liberation.

Five hundred years ago, Bhakti Yoga spread throughout India as a path to ecstasy and enlightenment through devotional chanting. Today, kirtan is still practiced as a traditional form of prayer, but it is also transforming into a new art form as it gains a substantial following among people of many faiths, ages, and backgrounds. Kirtan masters in America are riding Hatha yoga popularity to become a niche market within the world music scene, while the chanting expands beyond ashrams and into the mainstream. Bhagavan Das, Deva Premal, Krishna Das, Wah!, Jai Uttal, David Stringer, and Ragani may not be household names, but they form the music circuit that fuses the sounds and gestures of classical Indian music with the contemporary instrumentation and styles of Western music. Occasionally, yoga-practicing rock stars will accompany kirtan masters in concert or recording session.

It is easy to see the appeal of kirtan. Externally, the chants are simple to learn, and sessions can be trance-inducing, ecstatic experiences. The sets of repetitious sacred syllables are charged with intrinsic meaning in Sanskrit: manifestations of love, inner transformation, and obstacles overcome. A leader chants a line, and the group repeats, volleying the response and building the group energy to intense peaks before taking it down to soft valleys of serenity. Individual chants are repeated for at least twenty minutes, or for much longer periods. The mantras provide their benefits of greater well-being through *aavritti*, or repetitiousness, and through proper initiation by one in whom kundalini energy has awakened.

This unique manifestation of *nada*, the yoga of sound, becomes communal participation and an avenue for authentic practice. Internally, chanting of mantras as empowered vibratory sounds induces deeply felt effects, some say even if its participants do not fully understand their underlying meaning (although this point is the subject of serious debate). As Krishna Das once said, "It creates a sympathetic vibration in everybody, and everybody gets that feeling," like the warmth and glow received from a fire on a cold Midwestern night.[1] Swami Kripalu explained kirtan's meditative aspect this way: "The entire mind enters into the wave of rhythm and becomes one-pointed, focused on repetition of the mantra."[2] Repetition works on the energy centers associated with the body, including the throat and heart.

Is melodic chanting following the script of American yoga—changing and emphasizing the outer format and context while shifting away from its inner essence? Is it becoming secularized with growing popularity, affording opportunities for greater profits and entertainment? Is it just Christian Rock dressed up in saffron robes? Insightful kirtan masters familiar with both old ashram participants and newer secular audiences can help us find the answers.

## Chanting American Style

As the kirtan phenomenon grows, it also changes. Kirtan is where the music scene and the yoga subculture mix, mingle, and balance, where the sounds and gestures of Indian music are fused with contemporary Western instrumentation and styles. Kirtan seems easier to merge with Western music than are classical Indian forms, given kirtan's less formal structure. New styles of kirtan are evolving, being introduced and performed in America today. Some, like the work of Bhagavan Das, are devotional chants, traditional in intention and instrumentation and performed in praise of gurus.

Some kirtan masters like Krishna Das and Jai Uttal, who have the same spiritual teacher—Neem Karoli Baba—evolve a very different sound. When Grammy-nominated Jai Uttal performs at yoga centers with harmonium and tabla, he may stick to the more traditional chanting style, but on CDs such as his haunting *Music for Yoga and Other Joys,* he mixes chanting with hints of New Age, rock, jazz, psychedelic, bluegrass, and Indian strands. Others, such as Ragani, keep to a backup of guitars, bass, flute, tamboura, and percussion. Some kirtan singers draw upon Buddhist, Hindu, and South American Indian selections, as in the music of Deva Premal. Renowned yoga teachers like Cyndi Lee and Shiva Rea create albums sequenced to the pace of a yoga class, and they sometimes include chants produced by kirtan masters.

"In India, kirtan can mean a lot of different things" says Ragani, a newcomer to the national scene. "The kirtan that has been brought over (to America) is a call-and-response style of music. There must be something to kirtan if all these people—Swami Rama, Gurumayi, Muktananda, Yogananda, Satchitananda—were doing this style of music."

In many ways, kirtan rides the same balance beam as does yoga in America. But this time, the balance lies between temple and club, spirituality and entertainment, and practitioner and performer. Some kirtan is an eclectic "East-meets-West" instrumentation, at times given as much prominence on recordings as the chanting itself. Depending on the emphasis in style and instrumentation, kirtan has become a recognized current in the New Age and world music's ocean of sound. Krishna Das looks at the current scene this way, as noted on his Web site: "It is interesting to do it without copying Indian, to try to take the spirit and let it come out the way it wants to come out as a westerner, as an American."

Few kirtan masters have been classically trained in both traditional Indian and contemporary Western music styles. Some have a deep practice and connection to a specific teacher which has fueled their love of chanting and their sense of duty in bringing it out into the world. Daniel Paul, tabla player extraordinaire and producer of the CD *Between Two Worlds,* now performs exclusively with Jai Uttal on some 150 kirtan programs throughout the year in North America, Latin America, and Europe. "Among all the people I know, Jai has been able to fuse Indian music with Western music in forms that really seem to work," Paul says. "We are trying to reach as many people as possible who want to learn about kirtan, become leaders, or spend time with us in the kirtan."

Paul was personal assistant to the great Indian musician Ali Akbar Khan, having trained in classical Indian music for ten years. He also participated in traditional temple kirtan in north India, where it is a form of popular folk music performed as devotional music. In 1985, Paul began kirtan in Hawaii, and in the 1990s, he was traveling to ashrams, playing for free with a Western-trained classical cellist who was also a Vedanta scholar and composer. In those days, their audiences were typically followers of gurus.

Since the early 1990s, Paul has played with Jai's Pagan Love Orchestra, which produces that sophisticated fusion of Western musical genres with Eastern forms. Paul has also produced popular contemporary music, opening for Bob Dylan and substituting for his own percussion teacher in rehearsals with Van Morrison. Paul has seen the transformation of the yoga scene through his teaching with Jai Uttal at Kripalu: "I first went there in 1989 or 1990 when it was an ashram. Nowadays, it is much more of a fitness yogic facility with classes in some of the more spiritual pursuits. I think most attending kirtans there are more secular or with their own more personalized spirituality rather than something wholly dictated by a guru."

## Expanding from the Heart

Some Kirtan masters see chanting growing even more influential in the music world and becoming, like Christian Rock, one of the next music movements—and radio sensations—in this country. Kirtan's popularity has certainly expanded beyond the core audience of ashram devotees to a wider population through contact with yoga teachers recommending its benefits as a complementary form of practice. Paul says, "Some teachers bring different forms of spirituality into their classes that include secular-oriented students. A lot of these teachers are turning their students on to kirtan."

Teachers are recommending kirtan, because it creates an awareness of the subtle relationship of thought and feeling to sound. As Krishna Das noted,

> Any music that you do with passion and from the heart affects everybody. You know how you're a teenager and one of those songs comes on? The problem is the mental concepts behind it: 'Oh, my baby left me. Does she love me? I don't know.' All that stuff. I like to think of kirtan and chanting as those kind of love

> songs without the mental concepts, without the sadness. It's a different kind of longing.[3]

It is longing for oneness with the Divine.

Kirtan's central quality as a unique form of prayer and purification for Westerners may help to explain its growing popularity. "Mantras chanted to a deity are considered to be the subtle energy of that deity and contain his energy," explained Swami Kripalu. "Repeating mantras then purifies a seeker's mind and enhances his purity, restraint, and concentration. When such a yogi arrives at the source of all languages through mantra, he becomes one with God."[4] Kirtan offers such heartfelt intensity without sentimentality and the tyranny of neurotic thought and emotion. A repetitious chant then transforms and purifies the practitioner. "Kirtan is pure prayer," Paul says. "I think praying every day is a very important thing. To be able to sing and pray as a musician at the same time is a double whammy."

Ragani, too, acknowledges the powerful heart-centered impact of the kirtan experience. "I am not sure where the transmission of energy comes from. But I know one thing. I want each of the songs on my CDs to hold that energy." She explains the energetic magnetism in terms of opening the heart: "[Participants] want to find something that takes them back to what is true, to themselves, to their heart center. When it resonates with whom they are—something inside them—they want more of that. That's what drives people into yoga, too." Krishna Das put it this way: "Music is a way that we make love to ourselves."[5]

## THE KIRTAN EXPLOSION

Melodious chants' accessibility to the public means that some may be tuned in more to the music, at least initially, as entertainment. "Fifteen years ago, there were people practicing kirtan in the New

Age community that were not linked to any specific guru or set of teachings," says Paul. "Now that is much more prevalent. There are a lot more people coming to kirtan from a secular perspective. Maybe they're interested because of the spiritual overtones. But they are not as well educated about things as the older ashram folks are."

This expansion has opened up a completely new world of kirtan for the musicians, too, making it much more financially viable. The trick is to maintain kirtan's essence as it becomes a transformative form more suited to a contemporary Western audience reared on secular musical entertainment. Twenty-five years ago, the kirtan audience "was twenty- and thirty-something women practicing yoga who were part of the ashram community," notes Ragani, who played for Swami Rama at his Honesdale, Pennsylvania ashram.

> When I started, I wanted it to be much like what I experienced in India. But I realize it's going to become something different in the West, and it's going to be very powerful because of that. In India, the younger generation is hesitant to come to kirtan, because it's like going to church. Here, it's different. People don't know the mantras or Sanskrit or the words, and the music is a wide range of styles. I see people coming first of all because of the music.

Ragani took kirtan out of the ashram years ago and shares it with the wider secular community while simultaneously moving it into the recording studio. A close disciple of the late Swamiji, she leads kirtan at what she claims is one of the country's longest-running independent sessions outside of retreat centers—a monthly gathering that attracts hundreds of participants in a Wisconsin suburb. Such participatory music is rarely experienced in the ubiquitous sold-out arena concerts, and it is filling a void in urban communities once taken up by the youthful and progressive 1960s coffee houses.

Paul explains kirtan's grassroots appeal this way:

> People are becoming more hands-on, wanting to experience something more fully. Kirtan has provided almost a new folk music. It used to be people would sing in coffee houses or around campfires together. Kirtan picks up on that tradition and allows people to sing together again. At the same time, conventional music is becoming so commercialized, locking out young musicians because it is such a money game. Kirtan is leveling the playing field for anyone trying to get into a devotional type of music. It is so accessible.

## Maintaining Essence

The bottom line may be that kirtan offers an essentially meditative experience—sitting on the floor and quieting the mind to open the heart through chanting and music. This experience may differentiate kirtan from Christian Rock, which is more centered on the meaning of lyrics that praise a monotheistic being considered the only manifestation of the truth and the way. Yet kirtan can be threatened if its spiritual, energetic essence is lost through its recent Americanization. Ragani feels that when people get up to dance, kirtan begins to shift toward the nightclub, toward entertainment: "I want people to experience the energy and the music without the nightclub crossover. It becomes really powerful for people when they do."

The growing number of practitioners exposed to kirtan are traversing a trajectory similar to those exposed to contemporary yoga. As with yoga practice, the hope is that increased awareness means that more are finding its deeper message. "The practitioners who are older, learned devotees are never going to lose kirtan's spiritual essence, no matter how they practice it, whether it's fusion or straight kirtan," Paul says.

> More and more are going to be exposed to it all over the place. So it's going to increase the number who get very serious about it and pursue it more strongly in a more traditional way. I don't see it watering down the original practice, and all I see is a benefit—increasing the people who become aware of it as a secular art form who then may be drawn into it as a form of prayer.

Ragani concurs: "If it was just entertainment, I don't think people would be coming back every month."

Here lies kirtan's challenge—how to maintain itself as prayer once it is taken out of the ashram and into the world, a world that often just wants more entertainment. If Paul and Ragani are right, kirtan's essence and intrinsic power will ensure that it will remain a transformative pathway in the way Hatha yoga has an inherent ability to transform its practitioners regardless of their practice motivations. However, the danger is similar to yoga's—that a misplaced or misunderstood intention for practice will rob kirtan of its potential for more deeply transforming its participants. The challenge is to soberly walk its spiritual line while assimilating into our commerce-driven world, without falling to the side of either enterprise or entertainment.

CHAPTER SIX

# THE CROSSROADS

"Physicians live extremely unhealthy lives." The head of a medical training program at Walter Reed Army Medical Center in Washington, D.C., made this flatly counter-intuitive statement. She was referring to what she had seen firsthand: Many physician-scientists at the top of their profession endure unrelenting stress, have unhealthy diets, or do not exercise regularly. The program director was one of a handful of notable respiratory care physicians, among hundreds I met as a medical society staff director, who openly extolled the benefits of holistic health practices at a time when conditions for a yoga explosion were coalescing. Convincing skeptical colleagues of the efficacy of holistic practices like pranayama would demand hard empirical evidence. Otherwise, teaching pranayama to patients was not a viable—or even a known—option, despite the fact that regular practice would improve lung capacity, help clear the sinuses, and slowly address less severe respiratory ailments.

Some traditional doctors, like the program head, appreciate Eastern arts and sciences as they search for ways to restore health and enhance longevity. But what happens to yoga in a society that will repackage just about anything if there is profit to be made or influence to be extended? Is yoga in America at yet another crossroads, either becoming part of Western medical science or remaining a holistic path? Is there a middle ground, perhaps where yoga's spirituality becomes part of mainstream medicine, or vice versa? As described below, my interviews with prominent American physicians help to answer these questions.

## The Traditional Medicine Machine

Three overlapping motivations for practice contribute to the recent growth in yoga among the public: to get a good physical workout and enhance personal fitness, to practice as part of a larger spiritual path, and to promote healing and well-being. The last reason is most closely associated with medical care and yoga's potential role in it.

The allopathic viewpoint dictates health care in America. "Allopathy" is another name for conventional Western medicine, and it refers to substances, surgeries, and treatments that target a disease and create an effect different from the condition produced by the malady. Allopathy is based on the image of the human body as an intricate, complex structure of interrelated parts that functions to maintain the equilibrium that we call "health." When the structure is thrown off balance and diseases are diagnosed, common treatments include drugs and surgery. According to traditional medical science, biochemical factors influence our bodies and are informed by genetics and the environment. Primary causes of disease are explored at the cellular level and beyond. With few exceptions, the mind had not been given a major role in allopathic disease development, except for how our attitudes inform health decisions such as smoking or eating high-fat foods.

Based on this model of the body, the modern health system provides patients with mostly allopathic substances, surgeries, and treatments. Its hospital bureaucracies balance opportunity and risk. A patient's sense of self-determination, his fear and uncertainty, or her attempts at negotiation all intermingle with professional expertise and judgment, concerns for protection and compensation, liability, and malpractice. Hospitals—those caring institutions of vast technological strength—are the conventional pathways to recovery of health. Most hospitals have the same characteristics—rooms filled with sleek and sophisticated diagnostic machines, crisply made beds, a rotation of hoop-jumping specialists of all stripes, and charts of a patient's malfunctioning readied for diagnosis and intervention. Any warmth and welcoming is outweighed by the patient's immediate medical need and the system's assurance of a risk-assessed, probabilistic outcome. This home of the suffering, sick, and dying—this institutional oasis of mainstream care—is rarely a place of spiritual enlightenment.

Medical research fuels a multitrillion-dollar health industry based upon these systemic assumptions of body, health, and treatment. An enormous machine has mushroomed over the last century to include thousands of hospitals, clinics, medical training programs, research enterprises, and insurance and drug companies. Medical schools alone graduate roughly twenty thousand new physicians each year.[1]

Few of us would disregard the wondrous surgical and pharmacologic breakthroughs made possible through allopathic medicine, like "smart drugs" that target cancer cells. Yet the societal and personal costs of the short-term thinking in this industry are staggering. The desire to alleviate suffering and prolong life by relying solely on allopathic medicine's answers to health conditions feeds the billions of dollars spent annually to fund research based on this model. The critique of allopathy by medical practitioners and commentators has often focused on its narrow perspective or application, while, in juxtaposition, a model of global medicine open to other healing approaches has developed along its periphery. This is a natural development and a major source of dynamism in medicine because all systems of knowledge are limited by their own assumptions, including healing ones.

# Opening to Alternatives

Many health professionals today are not set solely on the traditional medical model. My doctor friends clearly do not fit the "unhealthy doctor" description. Professionally, they are trained in internal medicine, pediatrics, or family medicine, the gate keeping specialties of America's health care system, and they understand how a scientific application of anatomy and physiology positively informs the healing emphasis in yoga. In their personal lives, they are involved in Eastern alternatives—practicing meditation, t'ai chi ch'uan, or yoga while exploring the intricacies of the mind-body connection. They find that the major difference between mainstream allopathic medicine and the self-care paradigm, to which yoga belongs, is the latter's focus on the primary role of the mind in health and healing, on personal responsibility for one's wellness, and on optimizing well-being.

Over the past thirty years, the conventional medical model has been slowly modified to give greater attention to the mind-body connection and patient empowerment, with an expanded notion of optimal health.[2] Many physician-authors and medical science authors—Kenneth Pelletier, Joan Borysenko, Larry Dossey, Andrew Weil, and Dean Ornish, to name a few—advocated for this expanded model of medicine. Working with the mind is now part of the healing process in many hospitals and clinics nationwide that have embraced such resources as support groups, biofeedback, prayer, meditation, visualization, and even energy transfer. Research over the past few decades has assessed their positive effects, including meditation's impact on stress reduction, brain and immune function, and positive emotion.[3]

Family physician Zorba Paster, syndicated national public radio commentator and coauthor of *The Longevity Code*, tells me that "when we find effective ways to treat a disease in a nonpharmaceutical way, that is beneficial to the patient and preferable to more invasive strategies. Complementary forms of medicine like yoga and meditation are for preventing disease, and if you can prevent it and reduce stress, that's great. It's the non-drug way of reaching optimal health." Dr. Jeff Migdow is resident physician at Kripalu Center for Yoga and Health in Massachusetts. An allopathic physician trained in holistic traditions, he notes that

> the medical establishment and hospitals are definitely interested in yoga, but they are looking at it in a more allopathic way, with what postures to do for what disease. If researchers find that it is efficacious when used in conjunction with medication, it will have a place like physical therapy. So therapeutic yoga is very good for people to do, but it loses its spirituality. It is something else.

## THE STATE OF YOGA THERAPY

Despite greater openness to yoga as a therapy, the thrust of mainstream medical research remains the search for magic bullets, such as genetic treatments; experimental interventions; and better pharmaceuticals for depression, attention deficit disorder, sexual dysfunction, sleeplessness, and asthma. The profit motive, growing public expectations, and astounding medical progress are primary drivers of this search. That is why the Walter Reed physician's comments are so relevant. Trapped by a huge, expanding health system, many of those we turn to for medical knowledge and cutting-edge care are themselves on the same stressful treadmill that is feeding our need for the next bullet to relieve our suffering or prolong our lives. Some measure of insight and courage is needed to question from within a self-contained medical establishment successful on its own terms but seemingly unhealthy to many patients and critics.

This is the context in which healing yoga finds itself. Allopathic medicine, with therapeutic supremacy and widespread acceptance in

America, now places once-deemed alternative and spiritual therapies under its umbrella as complementary practices to be subjected to its research methods. Its scientific skepticism demands solid proof through experimental applications. It examines the Eastern healing arts through its scrutinizing lens, even though, prior to "medicalization" (i.e., placing yoga within the modern medical enterprise), many yogis considered measurable or empirical proof secondary to intuitive or immeasurable assessments of yoga's positive effects.

Consequently, the medical system can now influence changes in American yoga. Ramaswami claims that "it has become necessary to explain yoga in modern medical terms," as research is often funded by allopathic medical schools and through NIH grants. Coupled with the structure of health care financing, it is equally necessary to translate yoga's benefits into the categorical terms of allopathy for purposes of professionalism and payment. Ramaswami explains, "It is difficult to convince the modern medical system with explanations like 'energizing the chakras' or 'improving the *prana sanchara* [flow of prana].' With the necessity of getting insurance money for yoga therapy, the system had to bend over backwards to make it as intelligible to the Western health people and patients as possible."[4] In doing so, must yoga now withdraw central tenets of its worldview if empirical proof is lacking, since medicine's research methods are based on different assumptions about appropriate evidence and the nature of the human body?

John Kepner, Director of the International Association of Yoga Therapists, entertained in the December 2006 issue of *Yoga Therapy in Practice* the idea of whether "adopting the insurance, research, and accreditation practices of the larger medical-industrial complex represents a Faustian bargain or a natural, necessary, yet painful step." The answer depends on where we fall on the continuum between a more fully Americanized, science-based yoga and a more traditional, more esoteric approach to yoga.

Healing professionals working with the body-mind relationship have artfully integrated deeper yogic principles into their professional practices, synthesizing Western medical and psychological training with ancient teachings.[5] Through application of Raja, Hatha or Tantric practices, more people are being exposed to yoga's deeper pragmatism, whether in the form of physical movement, breath awareness, lifestyle guidelines, philosophy, meditation, or visualization. For example, medically trained psychiatrists with an interest in Tantra apply its assumptions to patient work. Jungian psychoanalysts draw on yoga's therapeutic insights. Transpersonal psychologists use yogic breath work. Allopathic physicians trained in Indian theories of body, mind, and spirit quietly introduce practices into their patient work. In all these instances, the line between conventional Western science and Eastern spirituality begins to slowly blur at the edges of the dominant medical paradigm as more Americans turn to these creative, holistic healing professionals.

Some are practitioners of *yougika chikitsa*—traditional yoga therapy—and use yogic techniques to treat health conditions. Traditionally, the search for ways to strengthen the body aided the adept's liberation and was key to the self-care and self-reliance underlying yoga as a path of transformation. The foundation of ethical precepts and observances, coupled with Hatha, all shared in the healing process and kept the student balanced and her bodily systems functioning properly as a prelude to progress through deeper meditative practices. To the extent that modern medical approaches to yoga for health and healing do likewise, we can say that yoga therapy's purpose remains consistent with the original, broader, and more subtle meanings of the spiritual path. To the extent that they do not, yoga and yoga therapy are more likely instruments in the allopathic toolbox. Therapist Chase Bossart makes the same point: "It is important to distinguish between adopting a system of knowledge, like Yoga, to specific contexts, and altering the system to fit into another quite different system of knowledge, such as conventional Western medicine."[6]

Yoga therapy as spiritual path—in contrast to yoga therapy as a medical extension—protects and enhances the traditional teachings while broadening their understanding and application. Ancient texts addressing yougika chikitsa can be found in the Vedanta, Samkhya, and Hatha traditions. Some modern approaches to yoga therapy synthesize these and remain based in traditional teachings. Integrative Yoga Therapy (IYT) founder Joseph Le Page grounds Yoga therapy firmly in the traditional psychology and philosophy of Yoga related to human health and based on an in-depth understanding of traditional texts.[7] The approach promotes compassion and well-being while educating clients, patients, and practitioners in Yoga's worldview in a way that maintains its integrity. In other words, yoga therapy depends on the focus taken by those who guide, teach, and heal. It can reflect either a psychophysical approach to healing, a deeper spiritual doorway, or both.

As yoga is mainstreamed as complementary care, its health benefits in increasing strength, flexibility, relaxation, and focused awareness are being empirically tested, and many claims are substantiated in addressing specific conditions such as back pain or carpal tunnel syndrome. With attention now drawn to its potency, some physicians and yoga practitioners see its mainstreaming as the natural progression of a previously alternative, but effective, modality. Dr. Paster puts it succinctly:

> Is mainstreaming bad? If mainstreaming means it's a mainstream therapy and it is a great idea and people enjoy its benefits, there is absolutely nothing wrong with that. Yoga becoming a tool for modern medicine is a natural progression. Yoga has been mainstreamed in many parts of the country for 25 years. Take the San Francisco Bay Area, for example. It's great that physicians are beginning to say, 'Go take yoga classes.'

Others might see this as co-optation, with yoga stripped of its spiritual, philosophical, and psychophysiological moorings as a holistic way of life just as it is happening through business enterprise, the fitness industry, and pop culture entertainment (without the influence of medicine). Dr. Migdow is well aware of yoga's therapeutic value for mainstream and holistic medicine, but he also appears more sober about the general state of yoga in America: "There are more magazines about yoga clothes and equipment these days than about yoga itself. The market makes what it can and then moves onto something else. I do get sort of annoyed when people make money off of something that is meant to be spiritual." In gaining medical legitimacy, is yoga at risk of being reduced to something it is not?

## A Bipolar Medical Condition

Georg Feuerstein, head of the Yoga Research and Education Center (YREC), argues that

> any efforts to squeeze Yoga into the much-celebrated scientific method is doomed to failure, which is not to say that Yoga cannot or should not be studied rigorously from a scientific point of view. In fact, since the 1920s various research organizations and individual researchers have conducted such research, especially medical investigations, with varying degrees of success, and their findings have definitely been helpful in appraising Yoga's effectiveness.[8]

If scientists respect the fact that modern medicine and traditional yoga hold to different worldviews and assumptions that are true on their own terms, there *is* a middle ground where yoga maintains its integrity as a spiritual path while its more superficial, more purely physical aspects can be assessed empirically. After all, the International Association of Yoga Therapists includes those who integrate holistic yoga's deeper teachings of the human body into their therapeutic work while recommending specific postures for patient intervention and research analysis. Empirical proof is likely to be less important to more spiritually inclined therapists who intuitively know firsthand that yoga makes their patients feel good, heals them physically and emotionally, and opens them to profound understandings about themselves and others. The opposite appears true for conventional therapists who are more firmly tied to the allopathic viewpoint.

Historically, medicine has been a potential avenue for yoga in America. Even before yoga became established as a reputable health regimen, its more tradition-based practitioners and therapeutic advocates sought to maintain its essentially spiritual basis. Vivekananda drew upon tradition, modernity, religion, and science to introduce yoga to the West. B. K. S. Iyengar used medical science early in his career to explain his yoga style while speaking in theistic terms about God as manifested in the *Bhagavad Gita*. Founders of new forms of Hatha yoga do the same. Postures, breath work, meditation, and visualization are recognized by more health and healing professionals as effective practices and as complementary to conventional science-based modalities.

As a result, yoga can be treated as allopathic tool for the therapeutic treatment of disease or disability as well as holistic path for healing while cultivating deeper sources of insight, compassion, and well-being. Perhaps the difference is a matter of both kind and degree. Adapting yogic exercise to medical treatment and diagnoses while strictly following the dominant medical paradigm is *both* related to *and* distinct from addressing the flow of life-force energy in exploring the psychophysical-spiritual roots of ailments while informed by Western knowledge.

## Seeking Common Ground

At this crossroads of science and spirituality—like the interface between holistic path and business enterprise—yoga grows in public and professional acceptance. It offers seemingly countervailing opportunities to *both* maintain *and* lose its deeper message. Since yoga makes a difference in practitioners' lives whether their approach is spiritual or material, measurable scientific evidence for its effectiveness under the allopathic model is openly welcomed by the yoga community. But even lack of definitive empirical proof for its efficacy would do little to negate its tangible benefits of well-being or its power to transform by removing obstructions to energetic flow in the body. This is not an argument for lack of evidence or New Age quackery but only a comment that empirical research is most appropriate and often limited to more tangible ways that yoga can be treated—as a set of appropriate asana and pranayama protocols for individuals with specific health conditions.

What ultimately becomes of American yoga continues to depend on the wide range of social forces that currently shape it—media culture, the entertainment industry, the growth of metrospirituals, the economy, yoga's evolution as an industry, the medical establishment, and developments in the healing professions. Regardless of which fork in the road yoga takes or if it forges an uneasy middle way, yoga's role as complementary medicine in America seems secure to Dr. Paster:

> I think we have to open ourselves up to Eastern thought and complementary forms of medicine. It's undeniable that the West has great medicine. You don't treat appendicitis with complementary medicine. For optimal health, Western medical technology has given us the short shrift, and this is where we have much to learn from Eastern traditions like yoga and meditation.

Kripalu's Migdow puts it this way: "There is always something on the horizon. I know that things that are love and joy will come and go in the culture, but new things arise that are exciting and interesting. So I look forward and wonder about what is next to come along for yoga. That keeps me inspired."

# Chapter Six

While yoga inspires us to maintain or recapture our balance and health, it also encourages us to train our minds and hearts as well—to take a deeper, more metaphysical approach to our transformation and to understanding our lives.

# *Part 2*

# TEACHERS, TEACHINGS, AND TRANSFORMATION

*As the wider society influences yoga, its gifts as a physical path can work in tandem with our willingness to explore its underlying promise—the potential to transform not just the body but the mind and heart as well. With the proliferation of teacher-training programs across the country, more trainees can cultivate their own innate wisdom and openness so that fundamental change becomes possible for their students.*

*The following chapters introduce basic concepts and principles that help us refocus the yoga experience on what are essentially spiritual intentions—to question and explore our relationships to practice, to understand how and why transformation can happen by applying teachings, and to learn how self-awareness arises in asana class. Our teachers are central to exposing us to the issues involved in learning to live Yoga.*

CHAPTER SEVEN

# Indian Interlude

As any gardener knows, it is not always best for growth to be strong or vital, nor must it complement the energy and aesthetics of physical space. In parts of the South, beautiful native plants have been overrun and undercut by a thriving kudzu that may appear elegant in its own way but which strangles and tangles more vital and cultivated plants. Similarly, the development of a fitness-based yoga over the past two decades does not equate, for some, to the expansion of Yoga as an ancient discipline and as a means for transforming ourselves when we feel lost or disconnected from our minds, bodies, or hearts.[1] Great teachers, whether from India or America, stress the importance of transforming this sense of alienation into a profound wisdom—a clear-seeing into our particular life conditions—and of transforming our preoccupation with "I-me-mine" into genuine happiness and compassion for the welfare of others. This integration, this higher sense of self, is the hallmark of Yoga.

By contrast, "small-'y'" yoga has more easily proliferated in America — like a transplanted, hybridized vine which rapidly spreads over its forests and grasslands, filling the nooks and crannies of industry, education, popular media, entertainment, medicine, and healing therapy. This development was well-intentioned. Yoga can be so much fun, can give us a tangible sense of accomplishment, and can heal and make us feel so good in our bodies. Those who feel yoga's effects are naturally drawn to it and hope that others can share in the same feelings of physical, emotional, or mental well-being. Yet applying Yoga to our lives demands so much more of us than feeling balanced or holding a casual, intellectual interest in what yoga can offer us. Our ninety-minute experience of Hatha yoga may rarely approximate the transformative power that Yoga wields for those committed to it as a life path. Yet it is where a deeper approach to Yoga can grow in us.

Consider an analogous choice we all have—the decision not to eat meat. While most of us would never give up meat out of habit and preference, some do consider vegetarianism for a host of reasons, much like their reasons for practicing yoga—to become more physically fit, to follow prescribed requirements for a particular health condition, to respect the sanctity of life as part of a more holistic lifestyle, or some combination of these motivations. The first two reasons are important, useful, and life-enhancing. Yet they are less focused on a broader and deeper motivation for vegetarianism—to respect and preserve life through empathy for the suffering of others.

While the consequences of our decisions might appear to be the same regardless of our motivations, the spiritual reason for not eating meat takes us deeper and becomes part of a wider examination of how we treat all living beings, including those we do not typically eat. The deeper practices of Yoga also become part of this wider examination.Vegetarianism and yoga practice taken up exclusively for fitness and health reasons are less connected to one of our primary purposes in living—to understand our interdependence with the world and how our actions affect the welfare of others. Once placed in this broader context, asana practice and vegetarianism both take on a meaning ultimately tied to the ethical observance, or *niyama*, known as *saucha*—the inner purifying of the body (as well as of speech and mind)—and the restraint, or *yama*, known as ahimsa which embodies nonaggression. Those committed to a more holistic Yogic lifestyle may typically do the poses with fitness and health more as unintended consequences than as narrowly predefined goals of their individual practices. Their primary intention lies elsewhere.

Like some practitioners, I am committed to living Yoga—this sacred dance—by coordinating mind, breath, and movement and by exploring its many practices. Yet sometimes, my yoga is just a vigorous workout more concerned with mechanics and accomplishment than meditative focus. This is a very common experience when we start out in asana practice, but it may also be where we remain stuck even after many years of practice. After all, it is particularly difficult to be brought up in America and not be influenced to some degree by the pervasive importance given to such ideals as sculpted physicality, technical precision, and personal achievement.

These ideals manifest all around us as TV and movie images, new products on shelves and Web sites, new services for our personal and professional lives, scientific breakthroughs in outer space and inner body, literary creation, and artistic performance. While useful in many pursuits, they also can be distractions or impediments to yoga practice if considered its main focus. When we prioritize these ideals, yoga more easily becomes adaptive product and innovative service—an ever-expanding, newly created series of challenging physical postures and movements and ways to think about them without properly maintaining attention to breath or relating the practice to how students conduct their lives.

Essentially, Yoga demands that we place distractions to one side. Yoga means acting spontaneously, in concert with the energy of awareness on the in- and out-breath. It means moving deeply in stationary silence from the sensory world. It is breathing in and out from the heart to heal. It is compassion and reverence for all living things—those visible and those invisible—and for the Great Mystery that is the ground of all Being. It is cultivating innate wisdom to find our own ways of acting from our higher self. It means holding to a stable love in an unstable world. These are elements of Yoga as a holistic lifestyle.

Practicing Yoga—like a commitment to preserving the sanctity of life through vegetarianism—has roots in a distant past and in a spiritualized culture far different from the one we inhabit. We might be tempted to draw close parallels with our own time and place. After all, humans throughout history have confronted the universal causes of their suffering—attachment, aggression, and ignorance. But these ancient people inhabited a world where egoism, ambition, and restlessness were not socially acceptable, a cosmos with a spiritual center where energies were known to animate everything around them—rocks, trees, mountains, lakes, the sky, the unseen world, human action, and divine intervention. This is the environment from which arose the great Eastern religions—what Westerners have come to know today as Hinduism, Buddhism, Taoism, and Jainism—as well as the inherent meaning found in the Yoga postures. It offers a worldview far different from our contemporary science-based, materialist one where what we know is typically limited to our sense observations and logical inferences, and what we experience is a more superficial and less energetic physical reality.

With origins shrouded in the mists of millennia far from modern America, Yoga no doubt spread throughout the Indian subcontinent because it was simultaneously practical and philosophical, grounded and mystical, offering a road to peace and happiness. While Yoga was originally planted in American soil as an integrated practice in the late 1800s, it would only spread into the mainstream of our society after it was repackaged as its more superficial outer form—the fitness workout.

Yet wherever it travels, Yoga's higher relief map provides tantalizing offerings—sophisticated philosophical views, or darshanas, informing our understanding of what brings a stable happiness, and detailed topographies as its pathways to that happiness. The latter include commitment to meditation practice in attaining inner freedom or release from suffering, represented by Patanjali's classical eight-limbed approach (Raja Yoga); love for the Divine manifested through devotional chanting (Bhakti Yoga); the repetition of sacred Sanskrit utterances with magical power in order to bring about transformation (Mantra Yoga); selfless, loving service as action performed without attachment to outcome, embodied in that Mahabharata classic the *Bhagavad Gita* (Karma Yoga); and cultivation of a discriminating and intuitive wisdom to discern what is Truly Real as found in the teachings of the Upanishads (Jnana Yoga).

Another form of Yoga, Hatha Yoga, offers realization through the physical body, with purification through postures, breath work, and the circulation of life-force energy, as embodied in the classic text *Hatha Yoga Pradipika* of Svatmarama. Hatha Yoga is the foundation for much of America's yoga subculture. In the traditional Indian context of the distant past, its tools were easily combined with mutually supportive practices like meditation, chanting, selfless action, and the study of scriptures, as they are today for the spiritual segment of that subculture.

These different forms of Yoga intertwine to create the multifaceted spirituality that we call "Hinduism" and to illustrate one of its fundamental insights: All is Brahman—Ultimate Reality. Their pathways to higher understanding address the varied ways that humans relate to the world—through thought, feeling, action, and nonaction—and indicate how we can learn to live more fully and happily and glimpse our true nature, whether in cosmopolitan San Francisco or sleepy Sheboygan. With roots firmly planted in Hindu spirituality—the complex polymorphous religion united by such notions as karma, dharma, prana, and reincarnation—philosophical concepts and mythic realities act as signposts that inform yogis' actions in this world. Its gods and goddesses—Shiva, Shakti, Indra, Ganesha, Parvati and many others—are different cosmic manifestations of what is intrinsic to each of us despite the fact that their names sound exotic or strange to those for whom yoga has merely been a good physical workout or challenging gymnastic practice.

Since Yoga has its roots in an Indian worldview sprouting these many practice traditions and concepts as found in the Vedas, that fact should be recognized, respected, and honored in America. These traditions and concepts intermingled historically with another strand of thought and practice, Tantrism, which is based, not in the Vedas, but in other ancient texts, the *Tantras*. Here, the focus shifts to specific practices for unifying feminine Shakti Energy with masculine Shiva Consciousness and for using the physical body as the mode of liberation or release. The Hatha Yoga we practice today is said to have evolved from Tantra, and they remain as both a method and a goal of unifying what appears separated. While most students and teachers may not wish to seriously study or practice Hinduism or its Eastern neighbors, they can still practice an Americanized version of Yoga that honors its philosophies and is informed by its deeper, universal truths that are in concert with Western religiosity.

To do so, we begin with the acknowledgment that it is the seemingly esoteric, hidden, or invisible side of Yoga that is central to its deeper transformative work. We learn through asana practice to open and energize the body. We work with focused attention on the breath to coordinate movement with the free flow of life-force energy, an initial gateway practice to transforming yoga into Yoga. We move deeper and learn through chanting and visualization to move energy through subtle channels corresponding to our physical form. We might feel energy centers open and recognize knots that block their motion and vibration. We may learn through meditation to quiet the reflective mind, opening naturally to an inherent wisdom that allows us to recognize who we are, to accept and love ourselves as we are, and to express that love outwardly as compassion for others. This is Yoga's—not yoga's—essential work, which initially requires guidance from those further along the path than we are, from tested teachings and practices that are thousands of years old.

In painting a picture of American yoga in the previous chapters, I attempted to leave my value judgments to the side, though they may have seeped through the words and portraits painted of what is confronting Yoga. But setting aside these measured judgments does not do justice either to my heart—my own practice and love of Yoga—or to the reader who wishes to think more deeply on these things without becoming entangled in philosophical nuance or foreign concepts that appear abstract or remote from their daily lives.

The remainder of this book forms a bridge between yoga and Yoga—between the fitness or exclusively health-oriented, asana-based yoga and a transformative, healing, and more deeply rooted one. In the first section of the book, the latter was treated as if it was one among many choices we can make in approaching the practice. And it *is*, relatively speaking. It serves as one choice among others. Now I wish to explore the freely chosen Yoga lived as a road to something deeper, and without abstract concepts that may weigh down rather than inform the reader's understanding. What is required is an open mind and heart. Without them, we cannot practice Yoga, only yoga. Without them, I would not have written this book. Without them, the reader should go no further.

So what must change in the process? I must change—from a detached observer to an active participant offering a meeting place for a more primordial Yoga and the highly popular fitness one—a sort of nontheistic bridge, where discussing classical concepts makes them more accessible and relevant and—I hope—does justice to their original meaning or insight. *Svadhyaya*, for example, was traditionally considered the study and application of teachings from the Vedas (literally, knowledge) to understand humans' true nature. In this book, svadhiyaya is broadened to include forms of meditation, spiritually informed psychotherapy, and mythic analysis that are means for transformative exploration. By giving attention to both experiential logic and to social circumstance, Yoga may become more approachable and less alien to those unfamiliar with it. On the other hand, it may lead to explanations not entirely consistent with classic Vedic or Tantric teachings. I am responsible for these inconsistencies.

In addition to my changed role, our relationship changes as writer and reader. How we approach and think about yoga and Yoga, whichever we learn to love, may also change in the process. We may be cultivating the ground together from which a more fruitful Yoga can sprout in our country, like the species of orchids in the gardens and hedges of south India—something perennial that is more colorful, engaging, deeply rooted, more meaningful to study, and more deserving to be harvested and placed in our homes and in our hearts. It is to Yoga that we turn.

CHAPTER 8 EIGHT

# TWISTED

Yoga can be a great workout. It can also facilitate healing. So it is not at all surprising that yoga's popularity as a workout complements so well its application as medicine—healing physical injury, managing pain, and addressing psychological distress. Yet the ultimate goal of the Yogic path is to attain a clear state of pointed awareness of the true nature of things, the True Self. This may seem abstract to some, irrelevant to the poses for many, or unattainable even to those who believe it to be the case. But such a refocusing turns us away from the pure physicality of yoga toward its deeper aspects. Just as there is a natural overlap between yoga's fitness and healing purposes, the cultivation of well-being through the practice of applying Yogic principles can trigger both a broader happiness and a deeper insight into our lives.

Shrinkage in the visibility of Yoga's underlying gift as a path of liberation—release from the broader human challenges that weigh people down—appears to be the price paid for yoga's wild popularity today. To put it in academic terms, it is as if yoga's recent "industrialization" is inversely related to awareness of its spirituality. As one increases, the other seems to decline. A cynic might recommend that we "just follow the money": As a general principle, where one finds exploding revenues and profits made from yoga as a health and fitness industry, one is less likely to see an authentic path for diving deeper into its depths. The extent to which we feel that this diminishes Yoga depends on our own disposition toward practice and where we fit in its subculture. Realistically, there is a middle ground that honors current economic reality and ancient purpose, integrating yoga's physicality with deeper practice, just as studios and retreat centers around the country are attempting to balance offerings of pure physical workout with those of spiritual practice and still do well financially.

There are Yoga practices involving loving devotion, intellectual analysis, selfless service, and meditative insight. They focus on specific ways for attaining release from suffering and gaining a glimpse of the True Self. They reflect our different dispositions for happiness in this life—the rational, affective, active, and contemplative.

Patanjali's classical approach, codified so long ago in *The Yoga Sutra*, contains the so-called eight limbs which today are associated with Yoga as a holistic practice in the West. These limbs or branches comprise Classical or Raja Yoga's methodology for transformation: making peace with our world through restraints (yamas) and observances (niyamas) that are ethical codes of conduct; cultivating physical health and vitality associated with asanas and breath techniques—the Hatha Yoga which is narrowly defined by many as "real yoga"; fully acknowledging our feelings and sensations while withdrawing the mind from sensory stimulation and interpretation (*pratyahara*); cultivating one-pointed awareness and concentration (*dharana*); developing and stabilizing that awareness through meditation (*dhyana*); and dissolving it into pure Consciousness—recognizing the True Self—where the distinction of self and other disappears (*samadhi*).

Asana practice, then, is more of a starting point than an endpoint on our journey. The physical and emotional well-being (*sukkha*) that results from it is a natural manifestation of this eightfold path, an initial doorway and prelude to deeper things. Many Yoga teachers may emphasize this point, since they are in the best position to do so. To the extent that we do not attempt to go deeper ourselves by fully applying the eight limbs, the more we contribute to the current trend that makes practice superficial. Our level of understanding and interest in living the path affect the degree to which we incorporate Yogic practices into our lives. This understanding and interest also determines the angle we take in looking at this issue and the conclusions we draw from it.

## Hatha Practice and Well-Being

Yoga's transformative work is not restricted to some faraway mystical level, and this no doubt is also behind its current popularity. It is highly practical and is concretely tied to the physical body, our interpretive intellect or lower mind, and the energy that links the two. In class, the postures work with the muscles involved in physical movement. That means that changes in the musculature of the body are a natural result of Hatha Yoga, and toned muscles are among its more tangible effects. Strength and stamina are increased while our attention becomes focused. Muscles, bones, ligaments, and tendons are strengthened and nerves stimulated through repetitive movements; the heart and lungs perform with better circulatory and respiratory functioning. We look and feel better. As breath work is added, students learn to regulate their inhalation and exhalation in ways that tranquilize their central nervous systems, build energy, harmonize the life force in their bodies, and (with instruction) guide prana along the central axes of their energy bodies. The mind relaxes and becomes steady, peaceful, and concentrated. We feel less emotional agitation. Confidence, a sense of mastery, and feelings of well-being result.

It is true that the power of Yoga is intrinsic to its application. During any type of yoga class, as we move in and out of poses, sensations arise that can be labeled as pleasurable, discomforting, and neutral. These feelings, tied to the central nervous system and energetic centers in the body, can last well after the end of class. They may be unconscious motivators for drawing us back to class, or they can keep us from becoming regular students. This suggests a central role of the mind in maintaining commitment and finding the will, determination, and love to practice. After all, where we put our attention creates patterns of energy that set in motion our cycles of habitual thoughts and behaviors (*samsara*), as portrayed by the film *What the Bleep Do We Know!?*[1] It is one of the Yoga teacher's roles to work directly with this mindful attentiveness.

One hallmark of continuing our Yoga practice through regular class attendance is experiencing some sense of progress. It allows us to explore what we feel is our limit, only to transcend it in time with more practice and without concern for outcome. If there are truly 800,000 poses and variations, as noted in the Hatha Yoga scriptures, then progress appears to be truly endless until we die, and that is the point. Since we are going to die, the ultimate meaning of our lives is contingent upon how we live them and the intention of our actions, including how and why we engage in Yoga practice.

Yoga teachings recognize the close association between our physical, emotional, and mental well-being so that "living in the mind," disengaged from our bodies and feelings, will ultimately spell trouble for us as we interact with the world. In Yoga class, a special reciprocity is set in motion between physical movement and feeling: Repeating the stretching of our muscles allows for feelings of engagement and relaxation and for greater blood flow; giving attention to our breath as we move draws awareness to the present moment. Coordinating the interplay of these physical, emotional, and mental aspects of ourselves through practice—feeling their synchrony—is one of Yoga's great contributions to well-being. But as important as that sounds, Yoga is not only about feeling good or being centered. There is more to it.

## The Asana Repertoire

Sitting, standing, lying down, and bending are what we do all the time. We live our lives by engaging in these common movements, from the first time we squirmed in our mother's arms and fumbled with her fingers. These movements are also the ways that we approach our bodies in yoga class. Missing from this repertoire of motion and position are inversions—which we rarely do in everyday life but practice in almost every class—and twists, which are so universal that they are part of every simultaneous movement to the sides and fronts of our bodies: turning to the left and across our computer keyboards to pick up a cup, lying on our backs in bed while stretching our legs to the side, turning our upper bodies to check for moving traffic out the side window, swiveling our hips on a dance floor. We are twisting.

Perhaps the twist is the most universal human movement or form of bodily expression. H. David Coulter, in his splendid resource *Anatomy of Hatha Yoga*, notes that fundamental to all twisting is the role of "torque"—any force producing a rotation through muscular effort.[2] All twists are initiated by torque, and all joint movements use it. As Coulter points out, twists are never symmetrical: they pull bodily parts to the sides in opposite directions. They compress bodily structures at the "axis" of the twist.

As we exercise our muscles in these asymmetrical and compressing movements, we squeeze blood from internal organs and improve circulation. When properly twisted, we move deeper and become more expansive in our practices. A key to our physical transformation through twisted poses is not to push ourselves and not to go deeper before we are ready. Our preparation—slow and measured repetitions with time (*abhyasa*)—demands that we strengthen those supporting muscles that allow us slowly to deepen into the pose, to hold it with greater ease and without strain or tension, to relax the mind with the breath, and to turn back toward what lies beyond us. To the extent that we can turn in time to see what lies beyond, the more apt we are actually to know where we are headed with our practice.

## A Deeper Twist into Life

So it is with yoga in America. Its current physical approach seems to be targeted at developing more supple and toned muscles while more fully relaxing into each moment of our overstimulated and stressful lives. The greater the commitment we have to surrendering to the physical approach as merely a preliminary step in our practices, the more we are apt to eventually see what lies before us *and* what we must do to go deeper in a metaphoric sense. The teachers who can best guide us—who furnish us with torque of another kind—are those who have learned to respect what also lies behind and beyond them in their own developments, including that which they have neither seen nor experienced. They support our deeper transformations—much like our muscles do in twists—when they point us toward what lies beyond notions of feeling and looking good through asana practice and even beyond any concept of physical or emotional well-being.

Feelings of well-being are natural outcomes of practice, but they become twisted once we assume that they are all there is to Yoga. According to the path, we are essentially divine—free, innately good, and self-accepting beings with tender hearts capable of dramatic progress in this very life. That we may not think or feel this way about ourselves is itself evidence of the twisted interpretations or labels we and others may impose, like leaves covering a diamond. Yoga as a transformative path helps blow them away—purifying and exposing us to a clear, radiant, and open diamond sky which is nothing short of an excellent metaphor for the True Self.

CHAPTER 9 NINE

# PROMISE AND FRUITION

*What thing I am, I do not know.*
*I wander alone, burdened by my mind.*

—RIG VEDA

The essential question of Indian philosophy, including the Yogic tradition, is, "Who am I?" It motivates serious practitioners to deepen their relationship to Yoga and means that yoga buns and strengthened abs are unanticipated consequences of practice, more than its intended outcome. Rather, the goal of practice—indeed of the Yogic journey—involves dissolving our clinging (*raga*), greediness (*lobha*), and aggression (*krodha*), which arise from our ignorance (*avidya*). Together they cause so much of our unhappiness and dissatisfaction. Seeing clearly is the ultimate aim of the Yogic marga, and using body and mind in synchrony involves practicing a series of methods for attaining release from our suffering. The physical poses are only one such method, whether we follow Patanjali's eight limbs or treat Hatha and Tantric Yoga as their own unique paths to freedom.

Chapter Nine

# Our Social Identities

In everyday life, we know who we are. It seems so clear. We may be mothers, sisters, ex-spouses, great dancers, Italians, thirty-somethings, Unitarians, office workers, quick-tempered, shy, cute, overweight, and ambitious. Social roles and psychological labels are the superficial expectations chosen *by* us and assigned *to* us, often reinforced since birth to help define and understand who we are. These categories can be respected, disregarded, or belittled, depending on our gender, age, ethnicity, social class, or personal proclivity. They are limiting qualities, however, making up our fluid sense of identity or who we think we are. They are subject to change even as we hold onto them for dear life as public personae ("I am a competent accountant who loves rollerblading"), defending against anyone who would argue otherwise ("She's uptight, nasty, and hung up on money"). We sustain or counteract these self-images, this self-importance and self-absorption, through our thoughts. In fact, by identifying with our thoughts, we tend to think we *are* our thoughts.

All it takes is a serious upheaval to realize the identity's ultimate fragility—falling in love, a parent's death, a partner who leaves, moving, going off to war, a therapeutic breakthrough, the trauma of ill-health, or the loss of a job that provided meaning. These upheavals are those moments in time when we are especially filled with power and potency, even if in the midst of crisis we do not realize it. We can open ourselves to whatever life will offer us without the imposed restraints of opinion or prejudgment. In the Yogic paradigm, a life's journey is millions of small steps on an evolving path providing opportunities for growth. Yet along that trajectory, there are places where growth spurts occur, where quantum leaps open our minds, bodies, and hearts to the strange and unfamiliar.

These moments are of different lengths, angles, shapes, and textures. Some ferment from the decay of lost dreams, places, relationships, and times. Others enliven us to feel we have endless opportunity. Some moments are loud and boisterous, while others are silent and muffled. It is in their spacious territory—at once unfamiliar and recognizable as pregnant possibility—that we can examine who and what we are more closely. For this reason, these are precious moments that ought not to be wasted. During such critical life situations and with some insight, we may experience a gap in our ordinary consciousness—realizing the precariousness of our lives and our self-definitions. These openings are fresh opportunities to explore who we really are, if we have the courage not to close off or shut down physically, emotionally, verbally, or spiritually. Their great gift to us is an opportunity to open, to love someone, to heal ourselves, or to extend a hand to the world in a meaningful way.

## Our Intimate Selves

Is my identity, my individual sense of self (*jiva*), real? The Yogic answer is, "Only relatively so," since identity is fluid and precarious despite what we would like to believe about its solidity. Is this all I am, a being cocreated by myself and others through language and culture, occupying this body in a unique time and place? The Yogic answer is, "No, you are much more than this." We can experience a deeper and more profound sense of self, one usually kept to ourselves or reserved only for confidants and potential intimates. This more personal identity demands genuine authenticity: an open mind and heart, honesty, and vulnerability as we share our deeper feelings, hopes, fears, and insecurities. Here we take off the mask and armor to reveal our emotional or physical nakedness. Feelings of tenderness may naturally arise, since we are sharing something truly precious with each other, more than mere thoughts or ideas. An intimacy springs from such critical life explorations.

Some of the more nonconceptual episodes of consciousness that we may experience—whether in birthing, dying, marathon running, lovemaking, enjoying Nature, or practicing Yoga—make us feel more fully alive and "in the flow," since thought is temporarily suspended. We may even momentarily lose that sense of duality, or feeling of separateness from others, through what humanistic psychologist Abraham Maslow called these peak experiences of life.[1] We might be left to ask whether what we experience—this intimate connectedness—is the real us.

Peak experiences, as sources of intimacy with our world, allow us to feel a more expansive sense of who we are, drawing on the universal energies that underlie thought and action. Feuerstein notes that experiences of *kshana-samadhi*, or "temporary ecstasies," are indeed intermittent manifestations of our true nature, according to an Indian practice tradition known as the *Shri-Vidya* lineage.[2] Feelings associated with temporary ecstasies are fleeting. When these instances are solidified or "owned" as part of our intimate identities or our running dialogues of who we think we are, they are not the True Self described by Eastern Yogic traditions, either. Yet they represent a fundamental doorway to greater realization. It is our challenge to surrender our clinging to any solid sense of identity or to any experience as some accomplishment, since they do not support the uncovering of our deepest Self and indeed can be a hindrance to its realization.

## The True Self

So who is the real me—before I was born of this body, before I learned to cling through my thoughts and actions to *ahamkara*, my ego-personality or peculiar identity? In *The Yoga Sutra*, Patanjali's first four sutras or teachings introduce Yoga as the process by which we rest and quiet the mind—our constant self-talk or reflection. We relax, let go of judgment and expectation, and release into our inherent nature—at peace. The True Self is the "Witness," Pure Consciousness, which is allowed to shine once we stabilize the mind. As we draw away from our fixed sense of a solid identity and stop reinforcing the opinions used to sustain it, we open to this inner wisdom which is pure energy. As Kripalu's Stephen Cope describes it, this Being-Consciousness-Energy is "the mind that sees and knows it all without judgment."[3] Its realization develops through application of the eight limbs, including self-study and meditation as well as the practice of Hatha Yoga—our personal laboratory for applying Yoga to our life. Yoga opens body, mind, and heart, releasing blockages to energy's natural flow as we cease identifying with our false or relative sense of self-identity.

The True Self is assigned slightly different qualities by the various Indian philosophical traditions. It is not a "thing" but rather is said to be clear, pure, unchanging, luminous, and nondual consciousness marked by feelings of bliss, freedom, joy, and love that cannot be fully described—like an indescribably delicious sweet, momentarily tasted in a peak experience. In the *jivan mukta* (the enlightened one who is living), mind and body have been tamed and purified, with their energies harnessed for personal liberation. "Who am I?" no longer needs to be asked nor answered. One knows intuitively. One is that—that which is Absolutely Real, Atman.

Perhaps the various Yogic paths merely offer us different perceptions and descriptions of the True Self when they emphasize consciousness of the Transcendental Self; realization of Universal Spirit as infinite and blissful; surrender to a loving, personal God; or the unitary Energy-Consciousness at the crown of the head. The goal of all Yogic teachings seems ultimately the same, and yet their interpretative meanings vary among achieving the Raja yogi's ultimate freedom (*kaivalya*), the Bhakti yogi's unity with the Lord (sayujya), the Vedanta yogi's release (moksha), or the Tantric yogi's energetic experience of unitary consciousness (*sahaja-samadhi*). Any commonalities and differences are a weighty issue of considerable debate and some amount of disagreement, which extends beyond the purpose of this book.

Yet we can safely say that awareness of the True Self remains the journey and destination on the larger Yogic map, whether practiced on a gym floor or in a meditation space. Its realization is both Yoga's journey and goal of uncovering our essential birthright. For the new asana student, Yoga is an opportunity to begin that transformative process by increasing openness and flexibility while strengthening determination and love. In class, synchronization of our minds and bodies through asana and pranayama is a foundation for practices leading to realization of the True Self. While most people who practice probably do not care who or what they ultimately are, the Yogic path cultivates changes in us just the same, often subtly, sometimes directly, if we remain committed to it and sensitive to its effects.

Yoga practiced over time slowly becomes a natural way to work with the "stickiness" of our opinions of body and mind, desires and attachments, all of which can imprison us in a false, relative sense of who we are and restrict our ability to see things as they truly are. That is why having wise teachers who have traveled down this path before us is so important to our development—to our blossoming as fully human. To paraphrase the *Katha Upanishad*: Being inconceivable, there is no access to this Ultimate Self unless taught by someone who truly knows it. These teachers remind us of the beautiful rose growing beyond our prison, if only we remain committed to dissolving the bars and freeing ourselves under just the right conditions for our innate wisdom and compassion to unfold.

Each moment, we are choosing what is possible for us in this very life. Yoga aids us in recognizing that we are that primordial Being-Energy-Consciousness, the fruition of its great promise and gift to us. Yoga means finding the Truth about ourselves without fear, fantasy, or distortion. Is this not more important than learning to stand on one's head, regardless of how the yoga industry has affected our perceptions of what is important? If we are serious about walking down this path, we must cultivate that which will fuel the entire process of our transformation—namely, the open heart.

CHAPTER TEN

# An Unconditional Opening

*Practice love until you remember*
*that you are love.*
—Swami Sai Premananda

Key to personal transformation and to sustaining a meaningful relationship to Yoga is opening the heart. Hearing that Yoga is about tenderness and the heart may sound strange to new students. After all, given the prominence of school, work, and planning in our lives, society prizes the rational, reflective mind in the form of abstract mental activity or discursive thought (known as *manas* in Yoga philosophy). Also, yoga is currently associated so exclusively with physical postures, regardless of how the ancient Yogic tradition points to the contrary. So how is my doing upward dog related to having that loving feeling? Sometimes I might just feel tired or irritable, and there are many styles of loving. So what could love have to do with Yoga?

## ACCEPTING SELF

Personal transformation through Yoga often begins with opening the body, which can lead quite naturally to opening the heart and mind. Yoga is initially about acceptance of one's physical condition and eventually about one's life situation in the here and now. Working with the poses may be our preliminary way to confront the fact that we may want to be somewhere or someone else, in some other body, or in some other condition. Through the practice and the initial surrender of the goal of accomplishing something, we can begin to explore who and what we are at this very moment in time. And with time, a loving self-acceptance can result.

In quieting the mind and synchronizing it with movement through attention to the breath (*pranasthana*), we learn to suspend at least temporarily the self-talk and opinions of others that we have internalized. As we learn to work with the life-force energy through asana, pranayama, and meditation practice, a simple realization often arises. *We are more than okay.* Our life conditions are fine just as they are, or at least they are workable. We are more than our bodies and more than our reflective minds. And it is the heart which makes it possible to go deeper and to discover the True Self. The *Mundaka Upanishad* puts it more eloquently: "Bright and hidden, the Self dwells in the heart."

## WAYS OF LOVING

Our outlook makes all the difference between being fully engaged in life and feeling dulled or deadened by its routines. We need look no further than to those who are deeply in love to find the ideals of full engagement and zest for living. Yet there are different ways to define love, and these vary with the historical period and the ways that our culture or civilization codifies them. For example, the ancient Greeks had identified many styles of loving, and contemporary behavioral scientists have elaborated on these over time.[1] Some loving is limited and constricted; other styles are open-ended and expansive. Perhaps we have all tasted one form or another and may not even consider the manic, manipulative, or obsessive ways that people express love to be love at all.

Consider these styles that originate from Greek thought as modified by contemporary writers: *Storge* is the love of best friends who grow in intimacy over a period of time. *Ludus* is the calculating, manipulative, and seductive style associated with the game-player. *Pragma* is logical love, where rational self-interest and assessment are key. *Mania* is that attachment-oriented obsession with a love object. *Eros* is the quick-hitting, romantic, and sexualized expression for that special one, glorified and sentimentalized through the popular media. Most closely associated with the love embodied in the Yogic path is *agape*, selfless love, where friendliness, compassion, warmth, closeness, and appreciation hold no hint of attachment.

Agape, the unconditional form associated with Yogic love, is egoless and applicable to all living things. It is commonly associated with the open, compassionate heart of the great religious figures around the world. Georg Feuerstein states that "ultimately, everything boils down to whether or not we love unconditionally. At least this is one way of describing the spiritual path."[2] Unconditional love is embodied in our own lives by those who place others above their own needs, desires, and interests, not in martyrdom but as a natural expression of their tenderness. If pragma and ludus are coolly rational, and mania and eros are emotionally intense, unconditional love is open, dispassionate, and free of clinging and obsession.

These forms of love are not always so distinct from each other. After all, we humans are complex beings, and we often exhibit more than one style of loving at the same time or may change our styles as we age or mature, moving from romantic to logical, for example. Some Indian yogi-saints have been well known for their unconditional love, and if only viewed from an external perspective, their seemingly erotic, mania-tinged devotion to the Divine.

## Cultivating an Open Heart

Unconditional love manifests as an awakened heart unattached to any one object, but open, generous, joyous, all-pervasive, and nondiscriminating. As part of the Yogic path, we can experience these qualities through deliberate cultivation. For example, certain Yoga postures, meditations, visualizations, and chants can be used to open the heart, even when we feel that we are shutting down emotionally or when the suffering caused by attachment has taken hold.

In the Indian and Tibetan Yoga traditions, unconditional love is ideally found in the teacher-student relationship, manifesting as devotion to teachers and compassion for students. This relationship is the catalyst through which students can progress in their love and understanding of Yoga as a life discipline. Therefore, finding a teacher who fuels her classes with an open heart and a commitment to a Yogic outlook and lifestyle is essential for being able to go deeper along Yoga's natural trajectory. This need not mean finding the classical guru of Hinduism or Buddhism. Yet a gifted teacher is an essential element in progressing along the path. Without a guide for a practice that goes beyond physical poses, it is far too easy to succumb to our deep-seated unconscious tendencies or impulses, known as *samskaras,* which derail our happiness.

Our ultimate happiness and well-being in life is contingent upon our ability to cultivate unconditional love. Yoga practice ideally becomes a safe container within which to hold and express unconditional love freed of confused intentions and desires. One of Yoga's goals, if we can describe it as such, is to keep the doors to our hearts at the centers of our bodies wide open from moment to moment and to place our minds in our hearts. As B. K. S. Iyengar has put it, "An intellectual mind that is unconnected to the heart is an uncultivated mind."[3]

This attitude of open-heartedness is not unique to the Yogic path but can be found in the writings of the world's great religious, mythic, and philosophical traditions, even those known for their presentations of life's meaninglessness. For example, French existentialist Albert Camus expressed the same sentiment in this way: "Live your life to the point of tears."[4] Live your life with incredible tenderness and empathy for life's joys and suffering. Such egoless, nonnarcissistic love is the foundation for a lifestyle that becomes a form of transformative artwork. It is the fuel that further transforms us to love ourselves and the world at large, to evolve from deadened and lifeless palettes to ones that are alive and vibrant with color and texture, in touch with life-force energy.

In the darker quarters of our postmodern world, this heart-centeredness is viewed as weakness. For the yogini truly dedicated to her path, it is evidence of insight into the essential meaning of life and of courage in the face of all that this world of negativity and cynicism, abuse and terror offers us. When a mind stabilized and focused through asana, pranayama, meditation, and chanting is centered in the joyous heart, we are less apt to become the Milosevic or Saddam of our intimate relationships, workplaces, and yoga studios. This union of fully awakened mind and heart is among the greatest gifts and most difficult challenges of Yoga practice. This is Yoga lived as a vital path with heart—a path of warriorship[5]—and which lays a basic foundation necessary for the discovery of who we are.

## CHAPTER ELEVEN

# UPRISING

Whenever we relate to others, there is the real possibility that we will change and affect the relationships themselves—how we value them, what we expect from them, or how we exude friendliness and create distance or divisiveness. Our openness to change, our positive regard for the other, and our honoring what is best for us in the process are the raw materials we can use in sculpting our relationships as beautiful containers of human creativity that hold continuous potential for real transformation. By its very nature, such transformation is not mere change, which is a universal hallmark of our human existence. Rather, it is a fundamental restructuring and rethinking that has a ripple effect on everything else in our lives. In sociological terms, this ripple effect is known as "resocialization," or the radical shifting of our lives in wholly new directions. In Yogic terms, it entails challenging what is referred to as our "lower natures"—our controlling and grasping egos—and surrendering to a higher, deeper, intuitive understanding of things (which yogis acknowledge as a sacred or divine wisdom).

Our relationship to Yoga—like that to a work colleague, casual friend, and life partner—holds potential for new direction and challenge as well as for the same old habitual patterns. It takes courage, insight, and compassion for us to create a truly transformative masterpiece worthy of celebration. The public's growing awareness of yoga means that both practitioner and Yoga are undergoing change in the midst of their mutual dance together. While this American love affair has the potential for a heartfelt connection, it is best nurtured by regular contact, the continuous spark of desire, clear intention, caring, honesty, and spontaneity. In this way, our relationship to Yoga can lead us naturally in a transformative direction—from the fascination of discovery to the maturity of conscious commitment as the basis for a radical shift in our lives.

## FROM FASCINATION TO MATURATION

The most important relationships are usually those that stretch and challenge us. They make us think, feel, and act in new or even uncomfortable ways—questioning how we present ourselves to others and what is most precious to our sense of well-being. We learn from them and grow within them if we are willing to take risks. We learn something profound whenever we open ourselves to an authentic interchange of mind, body, and heart. So it is with our developing relationship to Yoga practice.

In the beginning of a romance, there often is a euphoric feeling of fascination with someone or something new. The sense of magic engendered by emotional engagement, the excitement of new possibilities, or sexual desire means that we are seeing the other person and the relationship fresh and unencumbered by routine. Where love is involved, it is not a falling but rather a rising, an "ecstasy" captured by the root meaning of that term—a stepping outside or beyond oneself. Often, we may want to lose ourselves in that absorption, in fascination with the other person, and perceive and act on the basis of pure feeling with less regard for a circumscribed identity.

Maturity in relationships implies that intensity cools with time, that our fluidity solidifies, and we begin to relate to ourselves and the other "as we think we are," through the routines of everyday life and in ways fueled less by the magic of desire or spontaneity. Paradoxically, we evolve to become on one level "more real," with broader perspective, while on another "less raw" and perhaps even protective. Yet if we could remain at once integral and separate, intensely bound and aloof, and connected and disconnected, this dance may become a more conscious and fulfilling relationship. This also may be how Yoga evolves into a deeper, lifelong discipline.

## YOGA AS LOVER

Our relationships to Yoga may begin as careful, deliberate explorations to get in shape or to heal from injury. Yet they also can have, at the very same time, the intensity and openness of blossoming love affairs. With a growing commitment to the exploratory process—reflected in our motivations, intentions, inquisitiveness, and playfulness—our relationships can be enlivened to evolve with time. They, too, can become "risings up" to love as we explore who we are and gain the self-acceptance that is the basis from which trust, risk-taking, and openness can arise. Once the foundation of practice is stable, grounded in something real but fueled by that love and determination, our practice can grow into a maturity which maintains itself as an important aspect of our daily lives. Part of a Yoga teacher's role is to nurture this process in her students over time and to ensure that the object of love remains clear—the process of deepening our relationship to Yoga.

Here too lies the societal challenge for Yoga practice. If yoga is bought, sold, and packaged in so many different ways as a great workout for creating "body beautiful," it is akin to looking superficially at one's partner and stressing their sparkling eyes, physical build, shiny hair, or soft complexion. There is nothing intrinsically wrong with such observations. But if that is all we know or care about in our relationship to them, our connection is neither fulfilling nor deep enough to sustain something meaningful. It is not likely to be the basis for nurturing mature love.

As with a potential intimate, there is much more to Yoga than its superficial side. As with any initial fascination with the physical, our initial relationship to Yoga can become an entry point into something much deeper. At its center, Yoga is a discipline that contains the kernels from which we transform in ways neither foreseen nor intended. The key is to stay with practice; to keep going deeper physically, mentally, and emotionally while finding teachers and practices that foster joy and open-heartedness; and to find out as much about ourselves as we do about Yoga.

For beginners, there is no real alternative but to take the leap and test the Yogic waters to explore the options, much like those who seek a mate while remaining open and unattached to the outcome. Any frustration comes from attachment to what we think we want or need—in Yoga as on the dating scene. We may not have a large Yoga retreat center near us or even many studio options, just as one's personal marketplace for eligible partners may be small or may have dried up altogether. We may not have a chance to attend a chanting session or kirtan or to open our hearts to something or someone worthy of our love. But it is in the act of exploring that we engage most fully with both our lover and with Yoga—with our relationships as transformative conduits.

As with love, the leap into Yoga as a serious life practice is a rising up to our potential as caring, compassionate, wise, and wondrous people. The leap contains those elemental ingredients of love's many forms—desire, growing intimacy, commitment, and open-hearted tenderness (and I suppose, for some, even a touch of mania). Part of our maturing wisdom in that leap has to do with seeing clearly the relationship and what is in our very best interest. Part of growing compassion has to do with acting to ensure that its center is protected from harm's way so that it continues to be a trigger for continuous change. There is no one else who can preserve our relationship with Yoga as a transformative option. We have that ultimate responsibility, not our teachers.

When we feel lost in the deep, dirty waters of twenty-first century life, Yoga, like a seductive and dependable lover, will always be there to offer the way back to emotional, physical, and spiritual balance. That is its promise and its fulfillment for those who seek a mature relationship to it, fueled by love and based in truth. Ideally, we will find teachers who artfully facilitate and deepen that relationship with time.

## CHAPTER TWELVE

# Body, Mind, and Teacher

*If we wish only to teach poses or postures, it would be better to call what we do by a name other than Yoga.*

—Donna Farhi

Central to walking the Yogic path is finding a teacher who facilitates our growth. Despite important differences in training, yoga teachers share something important with psychiatrists, family psychologists, psychiatric social workers, and other talk therapists. They are in a position to raise energy and awareness and, in rare cases, even higher consciousness. While talk therapists focus on the mind (as Patanjali did in *The Yoga Sutra*), yoga instructors often begin with the body as a way to influence and understand the mind. Their students can benefit from the classroom application of Yoga philosophy and psychology, including principles akin to those found in talk therapy. Like effective therapy, Yoga class can be used to explore unexamined feelings and assumptions that underlie a student's thinking and acting. Giving focused attention to working with the mind and bodily sensations is helpful in making progress through Yoga.

All students bring to class a set of implicit assumptions about themselves and others. These assumptions are often expressed as beliefs ("I'll never be able to do that!"), feelings ("This is a waste of time!"), and projections ("They must think I'm too old and out-of-shape to be here."). With its initial focus on the body, Hatha Yoga appears to work less directly with these assumptions than talk therapy does. In reality, it provides many opportunities to explore these assumptions—while setting one's practice intention before class, centering awareness in the present moment, reflecting on sensations, and trying a new or difficult pose that elicits frustration or disappointment. A skillful teacher guides students through an asana practice, allowing awareness to emerge and, under extraordinary conditions, deeper transformation to happen.

There are some simple ways that teachers can elicit change. One way is to apply principles to class that are at once Yogic and therapeutic. For example, clients in talk therapy are encouraged to recognize hidden expectations; to surrender attachment to them; to acknowledge and honor individual uniqueness; and to take responsibility for thoughts, feelings, and desires. Such principles are consistent with the yamas and niyamas, the classical restraints and observances of the eight limbs of Yoga.[1] Therefore, it can be quite natural to address them in asana class.

## Recognizing Hidden Expectations

All of our interactions with others are informed by implicit but powerful rules. These rules—what social scientists call norms or expectations of behavior—influence just about everything we do. Yoga classes are no exception. Perhaps some of these unwritten class expectations are applicable to those you attend: "Please turn off your cell phone." "Face the front of the room, and sit quietly before class begins." "Keep your focus on the teacher and yourself, not on others." Still others are sometimes communicated verbally or nonverbally: "Come out of a pose whenever you need to." "Stick it out in a pose, because it is good for you." "Don't be competitive." "Let's see who can stretch the furthest or balance the longest." At times, teachers create these expectations, and at other times, students bring their own to class.

Expectations are so pervasive and embedded so firmly in situations that we take them for granted. We may become aware of them only when they are violated. While some rules are healthy and helpful, others are self-imposed out of habit, judgment, or fear of discomfort or of the unknown. Part of a Yoga teacher's job is to help us become aware of our unconscious rules. This process of challenging old ways of thinking and acting, embodying Yoga's rebelliousness, can provoke self-protection. Like putting on armor, we may try to protect ourselves against the vulnerability that new insights may bring.

Teachers can gently and tactfully offer students opportunities to examine that vulnerability and defensiveness. The beginning of class or during warm-ups is a perfect time for teachers to model openness and honesty by sharing their own experiences as students. Acknowledging that there is nothing to accomplish in class helps to frame practice as a journey that is its own goal, placing the issue of expectation or goal-seeking in proper perspective from the onset. Providing reminders while holding certain poses later in class also helps anchor the theme in students' minds.

All of us get out of Yoga what we put into it. If we practice to firm our thighs, we get firmer thighs through repeating certain postures. If we want to strengthen that once-injured shoulder, there are poses to help with rehabilitation, too. If we practice to become more centered, we are likely over time to become more attentive to the present moment and thereby more effective in life situations and more attuned to our natural rhythms. Yet it is through unanticipated results that Yoga works its magic, when we surrender or release motivations, goals, and expectations.

## Suspending Our Expectations

It is fully human to have expectations. What is optional is *dukkha*—the dissatisfaction or suffering caused by attachment to what we expect or desire. Once we become aware of an expectation, we can suspend it or surrender to it. In class, we may ask ourselves if we can give up an expectation of maintaining control and let things happen naturally, without imposing familiarity or order. To explore one's edge—psychologically and physically—means letting go of limiting expectations, not of common sense. The difference is key.

For example, a common Yoga practice is to listen to our bodies. This implies that we can distinguish between comfortable discomfort and unsafe pain. By recognizing the difference, we learn to hold a "comfortable discomfort" sensation, observe it without classifying it as pain or pleasure, and feel the sensation pass. That nonjudgmental quality allows us to release any expectation that things in our bodies need to be different from the way they are. We learn to "let be." Bringing students to this awareness is part of a teacher's gift to them, born of personal experience in the same way that teaching physical alignment is. When a teacher gently and occasionally asks us to scan for sensations and read our bodies' own wisdom—offering healthy reminders while holding a pose—they are giving us a gift of raised awareness.

As a teacher and student, there have been times when I succumbed to fear and did not even try to approach a pose that I expected was too difficult. At other times, I opened myself up to doing unfamiliar, challenging poses and experienced a sense of both mystery and mastery. Part of the difference was my willingness to suspend personal expectations of perfection and to let go of how I perceived that others would judge me. This is the type of personal insight that teachers can voluntarily share in class, not as a justification of fear but as a recognition of an empathic understanding of what arises quite naturally in class.

Therefore, an important part of a Yoga teacher's role is to facilitate this awareness-raising process. For example, when first practicing a pose like *hanumanasana*, or monkey splits, my Utah teacher's gentle and focused support made me believe that I could melt into the floor, without worrying if I could move into the pose. We discover something new about ourselves in these moments, whenever we acknowledge and release a limiting personal rule of the yoga game. That awareness often arises in retrospect and is part of Yoga's therapeutic value.

## Honoring Our Uniqueness

In working with their clients, communication therapists stress that each person has unique as well as shared needs, goals, and desires. In therapy, as in Yoga class, it is essential to become clear about these needs and not to assume that others know them, agree with them, or can meet them. Both teacher and student bring unique abilities and challenges to class. Creating a safe container that allows students to communicate specific needs or goals clearly and freely is important. Only then can teacher and student become true collaborators. However, once again, it is essential not to cling but to let go of expectation, including the expectation that the teacher is there only to serve our needs. Part of this letting-go process may involve teachers working with students individually to address attachment to the expectation that the class needs to evolve in a certain way; that students need to accomplish something; or even that their unique conditions demand special, ongoing attention. It may feel wonderful when it does, but it can be so even when it doesn't. This teacher-student interaction reflects an evolution over time of the teacher's role with her student—from expert to collaborator—and simultaneously of the student's relationship to Yoga—from "what one does" to " what one is," naturally relaxing into the present moment.

Yoga asks us to honor wherever we are and whatever we need or intend on that day in that pose. Sometimes we may feel like we bring a different body to each class. One day, we may be strong and relaxed; other days, we may be tired and achy. Whatever we feel is part of our uniqueness, and relaxing into the moment is acceptance of that uniqueness. One method some teachers use to increase awareness is to ask for a show of hands before class to gauge how many feel energized, relaxed, or tired and to repeat the question at the end of class. Another way that teachers may help students honor who they are and how they feel is by inviting them to draw attention to their Yogic intentions—why they are practicing on a given day—while asking them to match their intentions with appropriate levels of care and determination. Reflecting upon intentions at the end of class allows students to gauge any sense of change. Reminding them that this, too, is a letting-go of expectation allows spontaneity and uniqueness to naturally shine.

## Taking Personal Ownership

Why would we pursue personal change through talk therapy or Yoga practice if we are not willing to examine what we think and do? A last therapeutic principle states that we must take responsibility for our life situations, as teachers or students, on and off the mat. To that same end, some therapists encourage clients to learn and use "I-statements" and "empathic listening" to address important issues, ensuring that they own their perceptions, feelings, and interpretations of situations. This conscious commitment not to impose on others through the use of language also promotes egalitarian power-sharing. In turn, this engenders trust and contentment.

During initial centering in yoga class, students may be asked to close their eyes and to relax their minds, to suspend thoughts of past and future, and to bring awareness to bodily sensations without judgment. While practicing asanas, trusting where a teacher will lead us is a natural form of surrender. Many ongoing teacher-student relationships are based on tacit trust and understanding of that surrender experience. Teachers gently remind their students to maintain the experience by keeping awareness at the breath and not actively anticipating sequences or movements.

Teachers embody this surrender principle further whenever they "check out" hunches with students in class, showing respect for students' uniqueness rather than imposing interpretations based on visual cues. For example, if we struggle to hold triangle pose, our struggle may result from poorly understood alignment principles, injury, physiologic predisposition, personal preference, situational feelings, learned habits, or a range of other possibilities. Past history, of course, is key to knowing whether or not an assist may help. Only through dialogue and checking out can teachers identify the range of options to employ to help a student. This dialogue enhances both a teacher's *and* her students' thirst for psychological freedom by respecting their experiences in the pose.

When students are challenged to truly listen to their bodies, with regular practice they begin to see their teachers more as facilitators than as authoritative experts, despite considerable difference in experience and knowledge. Students learn to take responsibility for themselves and their practices through mastery as they are encouraged to check out and share their unique experiences of each pose. On the other hand, if students feel resentment for holding a pose longer than they want, that is clear evidence of externalizing responsibility and control while being unwilling to embrace their feelings—to "own their bodies"—and to release attachment to them.

One way teachers increase awareness of this process of "responsibility and release" is to ask students as they hold a pose, "Where is your mind? Are you trying to accomplish something in this pose? Are you surrendering and relaxing into it? Whose expectations, if anyone's, are you trying to meet? Are you listening to your body or to me—as a command or a suggestion?" As a later follow-up, I have occasionally asked my students, "Are you feeling aggression as you hold the pose? If so, are you projecting it inwardly or outwardly? Acknowledge what you feel, and know that you are in charge of your body."

Once a student truly listens to her body and sees the teacher more as facilitator than as authority figure, she has learned to take responsibility for herself and her practice. Both teacher and student have entered into a more mutually enjoyable, egalitarian relationship.

## YOGA AND HIGHER CONSCIOUSNESS

Fundamentally, Yoga and therapy are both ways of "unlearning" that induce healthier ways of being. They show us how to live more fully as less opinionated and freer people, with greater dignity and playfulness. By consciously engaging with these therapeutic principles, instructor and student learn to co-create a sense of well-being which can be taken out into the world as a model for living away from the mat. That application offers students in each moment an opportunity to remain open and unattached to expectation; to respect uniqueness; and to own and release attachment to perceptions, feelings, and interpretations. While this process only begins to touch upon Yoga as transformative conduit, it honors the ground upon which deeper practice can blossom.

In the language of Yoga, this process represents the natural development of *svadhyaya*, or experiential self-study; *aparigraha*, here embodied as nonattachment to expectation and outcome; ahimsa, all-encompassing gentleness toward self and other; and *santosha*, taking responsibility for our contentment. Underlying each of these yamas and niyamas is the notion that when our minds are truly at rest, pure awareness can shine through as "witness consciousness." When the mind is calm and synchronized with movement through the medium of the breath, nonconceptual awareness arises naturally.

A helpful way that we can work more deeply with our habitually distracted minds off the mat is through sitting meditation. Great yogis like Patanjali used the term *samyama* to describe the process of transforming the mind through sense withdrawal, focused attention, and absorption. He found that the basis for such afflictions as attachment, aggression, and ignorance can be clearly seen and, with much determination and practice, ultimately overcome. Regular Yoga practice—more than just doing poses—prepares the body for meditation practice and centers students so that clarity arises and invites the openness, empathy, and respect necessary for the application of these principles—the yamas and niyamas—to manifest. Yoga becomes our great therapeutic resource, sowing seeds for a change in awareness.

Thus, cultivation of Yoga is not done for mere pleasure or physical benefit, but for something much deeper and more significant. And finding the right teacher—a "transformation-facilitator"—is essential for the entire process to unfold. Renowned instructor and Tantric practitioner Rod Stryker tells his students this: "If your interest is in physical postures and techniques, then group classes and attending yoga conferences will be fine. There are many teachers capable of teaching those. But if you're interested in unfolding spiritually, you need that rare kind of teacher or guide who can reach more than just your mind or body."[2]

# *Part 3*

# Transforming Self

*This final section of the book captures the power of Yoga to open and transform us as we apply the practice to our lives. The concepts we use in the process are rooted in ancient Indian thought. As basic ingredients for our life recipes, they are more than dry, foreign abstractions. In the lives of serious students, these concepts—seva, shaktipat, kundalini, karma, asteya, ahimsa, dukkha, dharma, and many more—become visceral applications to our lives. Yoga's power, manifested in widened consciousness and an opened heart, enlivens these concepts through the accumulated experience and insightful teachings they embody.*

*This series of chapters represents concrete ways that opportunities for realization arise at different moments in time and in different situations: how meeting a very gifted teacher can deepen our understanding of who are, how chance encounters with people through yoga class inspire us to reflect on life's "big picture," how the powers of myth and of place hold underlying messages for living as students of the path, and how compassion and inspiration result from sharing in the trials of those situated on the border of our lives.*

*In all these cases, Yoga's meaning remains the same: As part of an interconnected whole, we are beckoned to explore the world through Yoga's power to open and energize us, and to transform within ourselves that which is dark, dull, or heavy into something light, clear and vibrant. These stories are offered with this essential teaching in mind, hopefully mobilizing the reader to consciously live her own life more fully and Yoga more deeply.*

CHAPTER THIRTEEN

# Zero Gravity

*Be the change that you want to see in the world.*
—Mohandas Gandhi

"It all started with loving and doing Yoga and then losing my way," Abby Lentz admitted. "Abby from Austin," as I came to know her, is a fifty-eight-year-old Yoga instructor from central Texas whom I met during my teacher certification training. Abby has since become an active proponent of Yoga's many benefits, offering online classes through a company that provides a "virtual gym" by streaming fitness videos viewed by students around the world. An avid cyclist and past member of the Austin Runners Club, she completed the famed Dublin City Marathon to raise funds for the Arthritis Foundation. Her teaching has been featured on the morning show of WOAI-TV, San Antonio's NBC affiliate. On the surface, Abby's is a Hatha Yoga teacher's success story, but her story's importance lies in the Hindu concept of *seva*, the compassionate and selfless service that it embodies.

## The Healing Power of Seva

While common to the various forms of Yoga, seva is central to Karma Yoga. It is working for the benefit of others without self-centered expectation or motivation, in detachment from the fruits or results (*phala*) of what we do. This form of renunciation (*viraga*) purifies the mind, opens the heart, and triggers our transformation once it becomes our natural, compassionate way of approaching the world. Seva is central to the Yogic worldview. It is found in Lord Krishna and Arjuna's dialogue in *The Bhagavad Gita*; in the Hindu epic *Ramayama*, where the monkey god Hanuman serves Lord Rama; and in Patanjali's ethical restraints and observances, the bases for living Yoga.

Seva can be collective, as in Pandit Rajmani Tigunait's rural economic development initiative or the work of the Seva Foundation in Berkeley, California. Since 1978, the Seva Foundation has served people around the world who are struggling to maintain health, survival, and community. Its principle of compassion-in-action includes building partnerships to prevent blindness and restore sight in Asia, Africa, and Central America; helping indigenous peoples of Latin America meet basic needs and create solutions to poverty and injustice; and supporting American Indians' work to promote wellness, environmental protection, and cultural preservation. Such service is global compassion in action.

Seva can also be highly individualistic, as it is in Abby's case. Portly, intelligent, sensitive, and insightful, she surprised me the first time that I gave her a goodbye hug, and noticed her size in comparison to others I hold in my arms. Was this a comparative assessment based on my experience? Certainly. Was it a condemnation of her 240-pound frame? Definitely not. Abby now teaches "Heavyweight Yoga" classes to other full-bodied people and empathizes with the feelings of shame that so many overweight and obese individuals have in attending an asana class.

Whether through collective action or individual work, seva challenges us to transcend our habitual concern for self by giving to those who suffer. While self-reliance is key to this tradition, seva ensures that both helper and helped become cocreating partners in its dance of social and personal change. As we actively listen to people, we deepen our understanding and helpfulness as givers, cultivate lasting relationships, and bring wholeness to ourselves and to those in need. These are the Seva Foundation's objectives and Abby Lentz's guiding principles. They are also the unanticipated consequences of giving, the reciprocal gift of compassion for those committed to the Karma Yoga path.

## Thorn and Salve

It has been said that in this life, everybody encounters some primal issue that is both thorn and salve—impetus for suffering and for growth. Some of us are stricken at birth or thereafter by disease or disfigurement. Some are confronted with lifelong challenges brought on by selfish desire, thoughtless aggression, or habitual action. Others suffer long and painful deaths. Still others experience a combination of difficult scenarios over the arcs of their lives. This is the mystery of karma—the extent to which events appear as surprising circumstances, sometimes out of our control but always tied to previous action in this or a previous life. Clarity of insight—our intuitive wisdom—spawns a basic intelligence within us to see the tendencies and consequences of what we do. For Abby, that insight was born of suffering and became the impetus for helping others who suffer in a similar way.

Abby started doing yoga in the 1970s, when she was a healthy twenty-four-year-old inspired by Lilias Folan on public television. As her personal tragedies and losses mounted over the succeeding decades, she began to "experience more and more stress, do more and more eating, and less and less yoga." She eventually yearned to return to the path that gave her meaning and to find just the right teacher, despite her growing challenges with weight. Abby traveled around Austin to take classes and finally found a teacher with whom she felt comfortable and with whom her weight did not matter: "Nina was my gateway to believing that I could become a yoga teacher myself without losing weight." Thus began a personal and professional journey that would pay dividends that she could not anticipate.

"When I was in teacher training, constantly in the back of my mind was the question, 'How can I translate this pose into something for a person with a body like mine?' It was my goal to bring yoga to this fringe group of people out there who wanted to do Yoga but would never enter a class. There are people yearning for centeredness and mindfulness who are morbidly obese." Awareness would become the first step in the magic that Yoga could offer to those whose feelings of fear and humiliation kept them from starting on their own paths of transformation.

Abby describes the process this way:

> Yoga's about the three 'A's: awareness, acceptance, and affection. In yoga, you first become aware of your body, because it is 'in your face,' Some people might think, 'She's 240 pounds. How can you not be aware of your body? It's so big.' But it's the same process that happens to somebody who is a size eight who wants to be a size four. They are not seeing their thin, healthy body as it is. They are seeing something else. . . . You're stretching and touching and doing things that you have never done before, and it makes you more aware, more alive. With that, as you gain success, and everybody around you is dealing with the same body type that you are dealing with, people find acceptance of their body. With acceptance comes affection, and then you begin to make different choices.

These are choices about reasonable amounts to eat; about incorporating aerobics or weight lifting to complement Yoga practice; and about integrating Yoga into everyday life when at home, when waiting in line, and when breathing at one's workstation.

Part of Abby's special gift is adding to the asana lexicon by using language geared to the overweight.

> I talk very frankly about flesh and fat in class. There's no mincing of words. I use terms like one's 'belly well' when you are moving head-to-knee between the legs or 'taking an energetic swipe,' which is moving your flesh away so they can reach their inner body and feel the stretch a little deeper. I want to create a safe place to do yoga where there is no judgment of the body.

This is a place where self-acceptance is nurtured to allow love to arise.

## The Weightiness of Yoga

America spawns weight-loss programs about as quickly and creatively as it does new yoga workouts. One long-standing and successful program, Weight Watchers, has led to many copycat initiatives that have as their goal the fostering of a more fulfilled and happy individual with a healthy and fit lifestyle. Weight Watchers' "Tools for Living" work with thoughts and feelings associated with weight loss. Weight Watcher members are taught to believe in themselves and their ability to change; to find inner strength and perseverance; to visualize the change; to identify stepping-stones on the path to weight recovery; and to work directly with positive feelings, intentions, and inspirational talk for reaching their goals and overcoming bad habits.

The Yogic approach is different. Abby does not calculate for students a magic formula of expected weight loss through yoga as physical exercise:

> Yoga is actually about getting away from all that. If you are constantly thinking about dieting, there is all that talk and judgment of success and failure about what you eat. There is never any commercial message in class about eating healthy or going to this or that place. It is a Yoga class, a safe haven. If you leave and decide to go to Weight Watchers, that's great. It just isn't the intent.

Rather, it is all about how Yoga's magic works naturally with body, mind, and heart to increase the "three A's."

Medical researchers on American eating habits report that almost two-thirds of adult women are overweight, and about one-third are obese.[1] The prevalence of weight problems has increased dramatically since the 1960s. Eating is a natural and voluntary act, so much so that those who are overweight can be more easily tagged by others—perhaps especially by the slender and fit—as having full responsibility for their conditions. As with reactions to alcoholism, some think the full-bodied who suffer from eating disorders deserve denigration because of that fact.

In Yogic terms, eating and other pleasurable bodily functions call for us to cultivate a healthy, responsible relationship to our needs and habits—purifying ourselves through proper diet guided by the niyama of saucha and moderating our sense pleasures guided by the yama of *brahmacharya*. Both niyama and yama work in tandem to loosen the grip of the suffering born of our clinging or attachment. Yet external forces, including the influence of advertising and our social networks, interact with personal feelings to throw that natural and voluntary action out of balance.[2]

Those who are overweight are easily compared to the all-pervasive, fit female bodies—slender and sensual or tanned and taut—found on magazine covers and in advertisements. Dr. Dean Lesser, a psychologist and Yoga teacher from Madison, Wisconsin, sees it this way:

> I have known many who are afraid to go to yoga class because of the photos of the 'yoga babe' on websites, in every yoga magazine. So far as many fit people enthusiastically show up there, there are those terrified to appear, because they are not glamorous enough. The main magazines promoting the practice give a very non-Yogic message while using the words of Yoga philosophy.

This is the basis for Abby Lentz's prickly thorn and healing salve:

> There are images that swirl all around us. The media, the movies, the fat person who is the butt of the joke. It's that outer judgment that becomes the inner self-judgment. It's not just that we can't look like Claudia Schiffer or the model in *Yoga Journal* issue. It's how we learn to judge ourselves and the people closest to us who have done the real damage, when we are growing up and called fat. It's a way to separate us out, and before you know it, you are doing it to yourself.

Layered on top of the psychological pain tied to fat jokes, exemplified by the 2007 movie *Norbit* and by a wide array of comedians' jokes, are all the commercial messages that promote food-craving.

The impact of these social and psychological messages follows both the full-bodied and the physically fit into yoga classes around the country. "When I teach one of my four regular yoga classes," Abby explains, "I can't tell you how many 'regular people' turn away. I can be in front of the room, on the mat and in a leadership position, and people will come in looking for the teacher, asking the most athletic-looking person in the room for the teacher. I see the disappointment in their faces. I can see the disbelief and can feel their resistance." The flip side of such resistance is assurance to those who are full-bodied that they can do Yoga in an environment and with a big-hearted teacher who is exactly right for them, so that they can learn to accept and love themselves as they are.

## The Reciprocity of Giving

"Every student is on a different path," Abby continues. "Yet our bodies crave Yoga. One of my students on vacation told me she did sun salutations on the beach—a very large woman in her bathing suit. She just wanted to experience the sun, and she gave herself permission, not thinking 'these people are going to be seeing my fat ass.'" Rather, she stepped out from under the messages of shamefulness and into the zero gravity of her newfound weightlessness, so that her heart could experience the natural beauty and lightness of the sun rising above the sea. She had learned through Yoga to do it for her heart, her body, and *for herself.* Abby's online work is also full of unexpected successes: "One woman e-mailed me out of the blue that she was feeling hungry and rather than going to the vending machine, she did deep belly-breaths. She just wanted me to know." Abby concludes, "I get so much back. My students are such beautiful packages, dressed up with ribbons and bows. They give themselves to me as gifts, and they don't even know it."

Love and freedom are natural consequences of finding the courage to walk directly into the fear and shame that holds us back from becoming who we are meant to be in this life. "This isn't like going to the gym or doing aerobics or jazzercise," Abby explains. "This is internal. It is your whole life. Yoga peels your emotions open like an onion. It can be scary if students are not ready to explore themselves. So they don't return." Perhaps some fail to realize that the very thing that they associate with their pain is that which they can use to heal themselves. We run away because it is too painful to walk directly into our fear.

Abby reminisces about her own challenge: "Taking that step. I remember being so scared to come to class, being fearful that I would be the heaviest person. It was hard at the beginning." Once she accepted herself, that was it: "This is who I am—the body I am. This is what I have to work with." Self-acceptance, in turn, is a requisite for the arising of love—"to love my belly just the way I am. I remind my students to be kind and gentle and supportive of themselves without criticism. They have been self-critical all their lives. So we don't intentionally talk about diet or weight. Yoga isn't about those things; it is about coming home." It is about coming home to oneself.

The yama, or behavioral restraint, of aparigraha embodies the principle of nonattachment or nonpossessiveness, and it is not restricted to tangible things. Yet when applied to experiences like eating, having sex, interacting, or other ways that sustain us as humans, it becomes a tangible reminder of how these experiences can easily be transformed into ends in themselves. As such, they may fulfill deeper needs for acceptance, recognition, and security, but they may be distorted as uncontrollable desires and seemingly involuntary obsessions. Aparigraha engages us to cultivate in ourselves the capacity to recognize this fact and to live more simply while turning our minds away from self-absorption and back toward what is essential for the happiness of others. This is the essence of Yoga as marga and as seva. With such clarity, we more easily see what we are meant to become—warriors of seva. The role of teacher is critical to our personal unlearning process and to discovering the Yogic path and where it can lead us.

CHAPTER FOURTEEN

# The Gentle Rebellion

*The oneness of the breath and mind, and likewise the senses, and the relinquishment of all conditions of existence. This is what is meant by Yoga.*

—Maitri Upanishad

"I do yoga to be more flexible, to feel and look better," commented Jan, my forty-year-old aerobic-loving friend, after our class together in our city's warehouse district. "I get impatient with that other stuff, that centering stuff." Many of us may be like Jan and practice fitness or health-related yoga. Yoga's spirituality may seem too esoteric or disconnected from doing poses. Yet Yoga's aim is to transform us, to simply guide us in living more fully and happily. "How does *that* happen?" Jan asked me pointedly.

## Yoga Pragmatism

As we have seen, Yoga is a practical discipline with deep historical and cultural roots. Even if we have been doing yoga for a long time, it is useful to remind ourselves how Yoga works with the physical poses, or asanas, which so many see as "real yoga." In doing so, we confront an essential teaching of how to relate to our bodies and minds, reminding us of Yoga's root *yuj*, which means "to join that which is separate." An ancient blueprint for personal transformation, *The Yoga Sutra* of Patanjali lies at the heart of Raja Yoga and includes the kriyas or actions that purify mind, body, and heart. *The Yoga Sutra* comprises some of the earliest teachings on the philosophy and psychology of the practice.[1] Jan was surprised to hear that Patanjali's second sutra or teaching translates loosely as "Yoga is the cessation or control of the swirling, reflective mind." She looked perplexed: "But yoga is about the body." Her response seemed so natural, especially if we associate yoga only with the outer forms we practice in class.

However, it may seem even more natural to identify with the constant flow of our thoughts, ideas, feelings, and sense-impressions (known as *vritti*). After all, they comprise our waking consciousness, which seems to give us a solid sense of identity. Our awareness of this mind-flow arose early in life, as we reflected on and labeled our experiences of objects, events, and reactions to them, through language. We each started to take ourselves as an object in the development of an ego or self-identity: "I, Roxanne, want a cookie." "See, Mom? I am playing daddy." Over time, our minds are comprised of impressions (samskaras) left by repetitive, habitual thoughts and actions.

From the Yogic standpoint, there is nothing intrinsically wrong with the reflective mind. It allows us to make sense of the world and to survive in it. Our rational minds and our senses of self are reinforced by many years of socialization, as we learn to filter, shape, and direct our lives through thought and action. "So how can this be a problem?" Jan wondered, not seeing a connection to practicing poses.

## A Drunken, Leaping Monkey

Serious issues arise once we live so fully in this habitual mind that it dominates as our primary way of experiencing the world. When that happens, we may feel numb, even deadened, cut off from our bodies (especially our hearts) and from our senses—hearing, seeing, tasting, smelling, and touching. After all, these are sources of aliveness and are tied to the organs through which we sense and feel the world around us. Our problems are compounded when this destabilized mind is agitated, reinforced through years of habituated reactions to situations. At times, we may feel literally out of control. Like the drunken monkey of Indian lore, we constantly hop from branch to branch, thought to thought, desire to desire, and person to person, clinging or sticking to those we assume give hope or pleasure and staying away from those generating fear or pain. Each object we confront in our minds and in our world is ultimately the same—impermanent and devoid of solidity. It is our perceptions, feelings, and interpretations of them that calcify and give them the appearance of being solid and inherently real.

We become those branch-leaping monkeys when our minds are not fully settled and synchronized with our bodies, when our minds are not *sattvic*, in Yogic terms—light, balanced, and graceful. Our confusion and mindlessness are fed by the mainstream culture into which we were born—its work priorities, its educational headiness, and its manufactured desires and entertainments. We might even feel that the culture's underlying intention is to keep us hopping. Mildly dissatisfied, constantly reflecting minds attracted by ever-changing desires are the global consumer society's dream come true. Such restlessness, coupled with our natural inquisitiveness, can be great motivators of both worker creativity *and* power shopping.

This constant reflection is promoted by the restlessness and demand for innovation in business and industry, where what exists is simply never good enough in a profit-driven world of ever-evolving goods and services. A CEO of a major international corporation described the current state of innovation in global business this way: "Everyone should be dissatisfied with the present situation. . . . That's what needs to be recognized by every individual."[2] If those who commandeer the corporate drivers of constant change, as well as governmental leaders, media moguls, scientists, and others hold to such a core value, it is small wonder that a restless unease infiltrates so seamlessly throughout the culture, to those of us who work and play in its consumer playground. Perhaps it is also why Yoga is reduced to yoga, a means for becoming centered or an antidote for stress, and why constant innovation is considered by many a requirement of successful yoga teaching.

So how do we stop jumping and sticking? The problem is not with innovation per se; innovation is a creative human trait. It is with the restlessness of mind, the ambitiousness without limits, and the motivation or purpose lying behind them. Such "busyness" undermines well-being—our sense of centeredness and balance and of what is most important in life from the Yogic perspective. As Paramahansa Yogananda once put it, "In the cave of inner silence, you shall find the wellspring of wisdom"—the road to our freedom.[3] So we might stop and ask ourselves: What is more important to us—ambition driven by an ever-active mind in the face of so much stimulation and mindless motion, or discovering a perennial wisdom (*buddhi*) that lies within each of us so that by quieting, focusing, and relaxing the mind we clearly see what is best for our happiness and the common good?

Yoga represents our rebellion against such a dominant cultural message. "Oh, now, come on!" Jan rolled her eyes at me, moving from inquiring to amused. Consider art critic Lois Nesbitt's story, I said, as captured in her article "An Insomniac Awakes." Absorbed in the busyness of the New York City intellectual scene, Lois Nesbitt admitted, "I had no real connection to my body." A creeping malaise and melancholy fed by her workaholic schedule, mechanical fitness workouts, and sleeplessness resulted in a life adrift: "I slipped more deeply into the life of the mind." Talk therapy did not seem to help.

Lois Nesbitt's transformation began with her first Yoga class. "By all accounts I felt alienated in that East Village studio: the purple walls, the incense and altars, the Sanskrit chanting." But something happened to her. As she moved through the postures, "bending and breathing and basically trying to keep up," she said to herself, "Welcome home." Later she would reflect, "The more I practice, the more I stay tuned to my experience, and experiences are gradually coming to replace opinions in my mind."[4] Ultimately, then, Yoga is a process of mental transformation, of becoming sattvic, of uncovering the wisdom to free ourselves from the trivialities and distractions that bind us in life.

Donna Farhi, in *Bringing Yoga to Life*, describes the transformation this way:

> At a certain point in the journey we can't go any further until we drop our 'I-dentity.' The mind that is defined by 'I' is also limited by 'I.'. . . This relaxing into consciousness makes available to us a new and altogether different view of reality. The energy that we have been using to maintain the boundaries of the mind and use the mind as a guiding force is now liberated to serve the unbinding of consciousness. When the walls of the mind begin to crumble in this way, a whole new world opens to us.[5]

## Our Natural Homecoming

How does this happen? According to Yoga, our inner wisdom energy is housed in that integrated whole that is captured by the term *shariira*, our psychosomatic complex of mind, body, and heart. To relax the mind and to feel bodily sensations, even for a few moments in yoga class, means that we are beginning to bring the "consumer mind"—a mind consumed by thoughts—back into the body.

Yoga calls for us to work with the breath to synchronize body with mind; to see clearly; to know intuitively what feels right; and to find our bliss, our dharma, the passion that gives life its meaning and direction. That is one way Yoga fuels transformation. Inner conflicts may arise during the process, as when we realize, "My mind tells me that I should not take that job since the salary is not enough, but in my gut it feels so right;" or "My friends say that I should pursue that relationship, but he feels wrong for me." While such circumstances are often the stuff from which the drama of our personal soap opera is written, they may also be evidence that we are beginning to recognize an inner wisdom, our inner voice.

In conventional Yogic terms, this energetic interaction of mind and body is associated with our sense of identity as well as with more subtle aspects of who we are. Through asana practice, we begin to work with closely aligned levels of self (sheaths, or *koshas*, described in the *Taittriya-Upanishad*).[6] They include our physical bodies of gross form (*anna-maya-kosha*) and our energetic bodies of breath (*prana-maya-kosha*), with their channels and energy centers through which the life force flows. By consciously engaging with our breath in movement, we are working more directly with these sheaths. As we quiet our reflective, processing, "lower mind" (*mano-maya-kosha*) through Yoga, we open to a deeper, more subtle body of higher awareness (*vijnana-maya-kosha*). An additional sheath (*ananda-maya-kosha*) is the subtlest body through which some blissfully experience the True Self. All of these sheaths interpenetrate each other.

## TRANSFORMING ASANA PRACTICE

Synchronizing our awareness with movement through the breath invites our asanas to become more than mere stretching or strengthening. It allows an awareness of energy movement to animate our bodies spontaneously as we take on the various forms. Farhi describes the process:

> This reanimation of the body cannot happen merely through putting the body in a position. Finding our natural rhythm happens through inquiry that is marked by curiosity, innocence and playfulness. When we bring these three qualities to our inquiry, we start to get more and more comfortable with not knowing. The executive ego begins to relax, and our external commands drop away so we can become receptive to the information coming through the wisdom body.[7]

For Yogis (as opposed to yogis), the body is not a machine to be pounded into submission. It is a form animated by life-force energy, or prana—that same force that moves our breath, consciousness, bodily fluids, sense organs, and our very cells. As we practice asanas while bringing awareness to the body, the life force moves in different directions to subtly shape the movement of consciousness. Giving attention to the breath in class means we allow prana to direct the breath. Calming the breath, in turn, gathers and centers dispersed prana. The poses embody the essential meanings of their natural forms of energy as mountain, crow, warrior, fish, tree, bridge, or hero.

Farhi sees a much bigger picture in practicing asanas:

> We are quite literally in the process of realigning ourselves with the rhythm of the universe. Having fallen out of sync with this primordial rhythm, we try to reestablish a harmony between ourselves and the world. This harmony is expressed when we can sit with elegance, stand erect, walk with grace, and lie down with ease.[8]

Postures not only restore or maintain physical health. They embody primal energies, as the committed practitioner is increasingly transformed to see herself as a bodily container of sacredness itself.

As it was for Lois Nesbitt, Yoga class can be our brief opportunity—a respite and homecoming—to return regularly to a focused yet relaxed awareness in the body. Like Donna Farhi, if we extend it to life off the mat, Yoga becomes a sacred practice in living and no longer just a fitness fad or wellness rehabilitation. It becomes *our calling* to live life more fully.

As we walked out of the studio and reflected on Nesbitt's and Farhi's wise teachings, Jan smiled at me assuredly. "I'll give more attention to what I experience in a pose and to when my mind wanders." For all of us, that is a giant first step forward into the deeper meaning and quiet cultural rebellion that is Yoga.

CHAPTER FIFTEEN

# Primordial Nature

*Passing on the knowledge faithfully and diligently is the duty of every teacher of ancient sciences like yoga.*

—Srivatsa Ramaswami

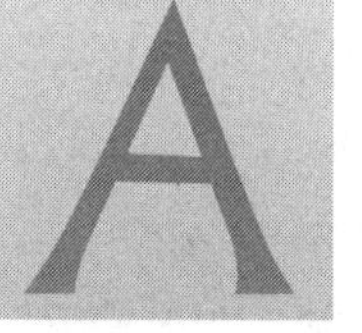

A few years before the yoga explosion hit, market research pointed out that yoga and meditation practitioners tended to be more urbane, worldly, college-educated, and female. Often professionals, they were health-conscious, loved natural foods and travel, hung out in bookstores and coffee shops, participated in the arts, and tended to be more politically liberal than the average person.[1] In other words, they were what sociologists might call cosmopolites—young, parenting, and empty-nesting city folk who appreciated diversity, who were open to cultural alternatives, and who often held more sophisticated and artistic tastes.

Today, big-city yoga teachers might still confirm much of the portrait painted by that dated market research. Students in America's larger urban centers can hail from all over the country as well as from Europe, Canada, Asia, Latin America, and Australia. They are of all ages and walks of life, many working in medical, university, corporate, and nonprofit fields. Their numbers have swelled with yoga's growth in popularity, even as the practice has opened to include an ever-widening group of Americans.

## Yoga Storm Hits the Coasts

Thirty years ago, big-city yoga in much of America was tucked away in funky neighborhoods, often near downtown or college campuses. It had an early association with things natural—bean sprouts, neti pots, massage therapy, and vegetarianism—and many things on America's fringe—chanting "Om," crystals, sitar music, and badly behaving gurus. Yoga seemed feminine, if not slightly effeminate, and definitely a fringe experience.

Then something happened—first on the coasts, next in the mountain areas, and later in the Heartland and the South. Yoga became popular to the mainstream and more than faddish to the fitness-, health-, and beauty-conscious. Still female-dominated, yoga seemed to explode by 2000 among what Paul Ray and Sherry Anderson describe as "cultural creatives," meaning those fifty million people in America concerned with such things as the environment, women's rights, and spiritual growth.[2] Now Generations X and Next joined those baby boomers with less alternative tastes and followed Hollywood celebs, rock stars, models, mavens, the chic, and the sleek to new studios set up to meet the growing market demand. Others listened to the advice of the growing number of medical professionals touting yoga's benefits. The segments of the yoga subculture were beginning to expand, interact, and coalesce in classes.

This change did not happen by coincidence. As we have seen, yoga seemed to be all over the national pop culture map, from daytime talk shows and film star biographies to movies and magazines. Yoga practice had become *the* hottest fitness and wellness regimen, with its own star power. It became the latest high; the sweat, smiles, and sensations; the way one felt after a good workout; and the way one looked. Books proliferated to meet market segments drawn to the practice—prenatal women, those recovering from injury, cross-training athletes, and even people too busy to find the time to practice.

Did something get lost in this popularizing frenzy? The thousands drawn to the Eastern traditions in the 1970s and 1980s—college-educated adults who explored their spiritual practices and some who spent years dedicated to them—no doubt feel a slow erosion of Yoga's wisdom center, maybe not personally but on a societal level. At the same time, they may have some sense of satisfaction as many more people have the opportunity to experience Yoga's magic. I am among them, feeling both the loss and the opportunity.

## TANTRIC ROADMAP

All of our life experience has an energetic quality, and Yoga is essentially about that energy—an energy of consciousness, light, and vibration that pervades everything. Some refer to the active energy as prana, the life force. Prana is inseparable from the mind—that which is aware—while it gives support to awareness. So it is said that he who masters prana automatically masters the mind, and vice versa. Others speak of the life force's potent, rarified form, kundalini, the primordial energy resting at the base of the spine. Such energy is intangible but real, experienced by those committed to the Yogic path as a serious discipline and lucky enough to find a gifted guide. It is best understood once integrated with daily life and can be transformative in its outcomes. Before such a transformation or awakening, life can seem dull, deadened, and lacking intrinsic meaning. Prana and kundalini are Yoga's liberating offer to us and its "super sale" to its new consumers.

Dr. Lilian Silburn from Paris's *Centre National de la Recherche Scientifique* has written scholarly works on Yoga and Buddhism. In *Kundalini: Energy of the Depths*—a book on ancient, esoteric Indian texts—she points out that "only an initiated master having a comprehensive view is able to penetrate the mystery and work accordingly upon the kundalini energy of a true and devoted disciple."[3] This is not the yoga done to a rock beat waffling through fitness clubs across the country. But it does highlight how Hatha Yoga, offering Self-realization through the physical body, is said to be an offshoot of Hindu Tantra. Both have as their goals the awakening of primal universal energy, and its unity with "wisdom consciousness" in the body.

Tantra Yoga is a particular form of discipline for synchronizing body and mind. Schools of Tantrism are nondual, not distinguishing between the worlds of matter and consciousness as Patanjali's Classical Yoga does. They consider the phenomenal world to be relatively real, as Vedantists do, while exploring how the depth and subtlety of our perceptions depend upon our experiences and assumptions, simultaneously as participants in and observers of life. At some yoga retreat centers throughout North America, these three philosophies—Tantra, Classical Yoga, and Vedanta— cross-fertilize and influence the experience of their practitioners (See appendix C at the back of this book for a list of retreat centers).

Tantra's nondualism implies that what is essential to every living thing—an energetic potency with pure awareness—also exists in every cell of our bodies and in every molecule of the universe. Coming to this fundamental realization in this body and in this life is a liberation to which Hindu Tantra students or tantrikas aspire through coordinated practices: asana and pranayama; mantra chanting and kriyas, or acts of cleansing; mudras, or sacred gestures; *pujas*, or forms of deity worship; and visualizations and meditations. Performing these practices stills the reflective mind, balances the subtle life force, awakens dormant energy, and assures its freed flow throughout the body.

Working with every experience we have means none are rejected out of hand since every thought and feeling is accompanied by a corresponding energetic character and vibration. This creative energy-consciousness unfolds throughout the entire world, which is apprehended as wondrous, pulsating, and inherently beautiful. Its potency is pure desire from the Tantric point of view. Daniel Odier, author of *Desire: The Tantric Path to Awakening*, notes that "each contact with reality becomes a celebration of the universality of desire" for the tantrika.[4] Just as desire moves the flower to open to the sun, it draws humans to manifest their true nature. This pure or higher desire is not our petty hunger to possess objects. As Rammurti Mishra defines it, Yoga itself is "submission of lower desire to higher desire."[5] Shariira, or our mind-body-heart complex, when balanced and synchronized with awareness, is the vehicle for that transformation.

## Mysticism as Transformation

I am blessed to know some of these truths firsthand.[6] As a fifty-something baby boom professional, a spiritual shopper from the 1970s and 1980s, I practiced yoga and meditation for years, occasionally taking a class here or there. Then, at the time when yoga was taking off as the next hot product, I met a teacher who taught Yoga at a storefront Buddhist meditation center. She would become a conduit for my own transformation.

I had never met an instructor quite like Sylvie Horvath. Outwardly, she seemed to be a typical yoga teacher—a slender, confident, highly flexible, and pretty woman. Yet she also seemed a bit otherworldly, quiet, humble, unconcerned with trivialities, and focused on what is essential to Yoga—on love and Self-awareness. Her talks at the beginning of class often focused on the nature of our false selves or identities and on how Yoga was the means for piercing their ultimate unreality. Her classes were different, indeed, from my experience of classes around the country.

Sylvie grew up in Nevada and took up yoga at age sixteen. She lived at ashrams in India, involved with two Hindu masters of the Sacha Baba lineage. On one of her frequent trips to North India, she declined an opportunity to join their order as a teaching swami.

She also had met with Sri Swami Nagananda in South India who suggested that she be initiated into *his* order as a swami. Sylvie again declined, as she explains it, wanting to live the householder life in America. Still later, she trained at Amrit Desai's Yoga Institute in Salt Springs, Florida. She now maintains regular contacts in India for both spiritual and business reasons, as she runs her Jewel of India import firm.

In 1989, Sylvie settled with her husband on Milwaukee's east side near Lake Michigan and began teaching. "The yoga scene was relatively nonexistent back then," she says. "There were one or two studios that I was aware of. Not many people knew much about Yoga."

Her classes are an eclectic mix of philosophy, meditation, poses, breath work, chanting, and visualization. Having practiced now for twenty-five years, she says students often discover that Yoga gives them a "self-awareness which makes them curious to know more. They develop a keener awareness of the deeper truths about life, the beauty of life, and their part in it." This yogini was definitely not a spandex devotee of the yoga explosion or some ordinary priestess-in-training, as I would learn.

Within two years of Yoga practice with Sylvie three times a week, I began to feel a growing joy and happiness that can best be called love, as if my heart was pulled out of my chest and exposed to sunlight. I also began to feel my energy centers open—first those above my heart—while synchronizing my breath with movement in the poses. With time, I became more proficient in applying the physical locks or *bhandhas* in class that open the flow of energy, in chanting, and in holding the visualizations Sylvie taught.

I enthusiastically started regular pranayama, visualization, and meditation practice at home, keenly aware of the new sensations—*prana-utthana*, or pranic awakenings—I began experiencing along my spine, first at the higher energy centers and especially in my frontal lobe. The practices, or sadhanas, Sylvie taught eventually became routine and daily. I soon realized that I was not alone, as other dedicated students discussed their experiences of prana with me after class.

While seated at home in easy pose or *sukhasana* on a meditation cushion, I would begin breathing in and out slowly, maintaining *ujayi* or ocean-sounding breath throughout my morning or evening practice. I then moved into three rounds of *kapalabhati*, or skull shining breath. These were followed by breath retention in *agni saur dhauti* (or fire wash) and in *ashvini mudra* (or horsetail) that involve bhandhas at the throat, abdomen, perineum, and sphincter muscle. With eyes lifted upward and slightly closed in a gesture known as *shambhavi mudra*, I would perform *nadi shodhana* or alternate nostril breathing that led into formless meditation practice. All I knew was that I felt good, more alert and conscious, more alive and joyous, and that I was not pursuing any conscious end through these practices.

Like so many Yoga practitioners before me, I was engaging directly with prana in the central channel of my subtle body. I chanted the *bija* mantra "seed syllables" associated with the energy centers while visualizing the energy as brilliant white light moving up and down the central channel. By employing *antah trataka*, I gazed at the energy centers' representation (*akshara*) on a page and then closed my eyes to visualize the same object at the appropriate center in my body. I ended the practice by chanting the *omkari japa* and sending bursts of energy from *anahata*, or the heart center, to my teacher and to all beings, thereby dedicating the merit (*punya*)—the accumulated benefit—of my practice. During these sitting periods, I would feel waves of pleasurable sensations with movement of the breath, and they often spontaneously returned during my workday and in the evening. Eventually, merely shifting awareness to *ajna* chakra between my eyebrows would occasionally open that energy center.

Unexpectedly, I began to have experiences that I intuitively knew were associated with Yoga and with my apprenticeship to Sylvie. I realized that she had a penchant for reading my mind, which became a common occurrence as I questioned her on the finer points of practice and philosophy. At home one evening, I felt as if my mind was being pulled right out of my skull, like the Vulcan mind-meld on the old *Star Trek* series and perhaps like what some term the "mixing of mind and guru." My first reaction was "Whoa, hold on!" because it scared me. So I chanted to calm and protect myself. Another night, I awoke to feel my energy centers being cleansed from bottom to top, a subtle but real experience.

In my concern to understand these experiences, I turned to the late Lama Karma Jinpa Zangpo—an affable, gentle, and insightful monk-acquaintance of mine who was associated with the local Shambhala Center. Lama Jinpa was an American and an ex-musician from the Boston area who had initially studied Hinduism and who maintained close ties to an elderly Hindu monk out East. He gravitated toward Buddhism and eventually took vows to become a monk himself in a Tibetan lineage. Over lunch at a Chinese restaurant, he affirmed for me the close correspondence between esoteric Hindu and Buddhist descriptions of the ultimate nature of things. He also confirmed that my description of the cleansing of the chakras was identical to how it was described in Tantric Buddhist texts—from bottom to top. He recommended that I dedicate whatever I experience to the benefit of all beings.

On yet another night, I awoke out of a dream to feel heat and then a burning sensation spread from my solar plexus upward over my chest. *Tapas*—one of the niyamas, or behavioral observances, of Patanjali's Classical Yoga—comes from the root *tap*, meaning "to burn," and is most often associated with the determination (*vyayama*), discipline (*atma-nigraha*), enthusiasm, love, and even austerities needed to progress along the Yogic path. In closing my eyes, I had a vision. I was a baby in diapers seated on the floor. My pudgy legs and hands extended out before me, with a block and a ball in front of me. This was not a dream. This was *me*, and these were my toys long ago. My sense of identity was beginning to expand to encompass my past more fully and consciously, embracing it as part of the Yogic journey. When I thought about it later, it occurred to me that this deep-seated, latent impression (*vasana*), must be tied to some early emotional experience.

These experiences were certainly out of the ordinary. But others, like the bliss of "a thousand pin pricks of pleasure" showering down my frontal lobe, became more commonplace. With time and further reflection, I would consider all these experiences Yogic purifications written about in ancient texts. They are all preparations, all signposts to go deeper in the direction of who I truly am—somewhere a popularized yoga workout could never take me. As Georg Feuerstein has explained, "The Yogic path can be viewed as a lengthy process of physical and mental purification."[7] Yet I knew these experiences had been possible only through the power inherent in the relationship with my teacher.

## Demystifying the Mystifying

While there are many Hindu and Buddhist Tantric schools, one explanation of paranormal or mystical experiences is that they result from the opening and closing of energy points in our bodies through Yogic practices. Perhaps my most profound experience was the one that took place on an early November morning. Shortly after waking, I was seated in front of my computer when I felt a slow-growing sensation that blossomed into the most intense pleasure that I have ever experienced in my body. It was nothing short of a spiritual orgasm but without erection, ejaculation, or any object of pleasure. It was the pure intense kundalini energy experienced as nondual pleasure at my second chakra, *svadhisthana*, one of the swirling energy vortices of human beings' subtle bodies, according to Yoga physiology. But there was *always* an object of pleasure, I reasoned afterward. Why was there none with this experience?

According to Hindu Tantra, our "energy-minds" naturally draw to places in the body and to life situations that call for healing.

Yet I knew this blissful experience meant much more than some intense, uncommon experience. I called Sylvie, and she picked up the phone with an enigmatic "Tom, I hope you have something juicy to tell me." Later, in a more sober moment, she challenged me to "recognize it for what it is. You *are* that energy"—that same potent energy permeating everybody and everything. After I described my experience to Lama Jinpa and sought his wise counsel, he advised me in deadpan style, "Maybe you should be careful where you put your mind"—good advice, since the second energy center is associated with afflictive emotions, often overwhelming desire, as well as potency, insight, and creativity. As the Buddhist Tantra master Lama Yeshe once said, "The essence of tantra is dealing skillfully with pleasure,"[8] with that pure energy and desire so essential to all our forms of creative expression and communication.

These are transformative aspects of Yoga that remain on the fringe of its current boom in popularity. As Silburn says, the ancient Indian texts of the Kaula, Trika, and Krana schools (as well as others) preserve the teachings and practices of Yoga's esoteric core. To serious practitioners, kundalini energy is the universal, conscious, and potent energy manifested as rhythmic vibration; it is ungraspable and ultimately indescribable through language. Kundalini energy cannot be anticipated or controlled. It is a source for both the expansive and vital life-force energy and *virya*, or the virile and potent aspect of energetic intensity.

Kundalini flows up the central energy channel (*nadi sushumna*) through the energy centers of the subtle body. It can reach the crown chakra (*sahasrara*) at the top of the head. But that is a very rare achievement, even for those devoted to Tantra over a lifetime. The movement of kundalini demands a cultivated ability to stabilize the mind-energy in Sushumna—the central nadi, or channel—and not to consciously direct or allow it to be drawn to any particular chakra. Calling the movement of kundalini to the crown chakra "the ultimate achievement on the path of energy," Silburn explains that "a prerequisite is for the yogi to be naturally centered in the heart."[9] This energy movement calls for authentic cultivation of *sahrdaya*, a vibrant, awakened heart which spontaneously transmits its power to the other centers. One would be hard-pressed to find fitness yoga classes that give primacy to centering one's attention in the tender, open heart.

Through initiations, highly skilled teachers with clear intention and knowledge use their own kundalini to enter the student's body and pierce its energy centers that allow him to experience some of the effects of the ascent of kundalini, symbolically embodied in the form of the Goddess Shakti. The initiations are also used by some teachers as a kind of spiritual "shock and awe," jarring the student into a more accurate perception of reality by freeing him from the prison of his ordinary, reflective mind.

The initiation is referred to as *Shaktipat.* Given its potency, this aspect of practice remains secretive and is reserved for dedicated students, in order to preserve its essential meaning and transformative power. In the wrong hands, Shaktipat can have dangerous consequences and may sidetrack one into grasping after such experiences as the goal of practice. Through Shaktipat, passive descent of wisdom consciousness meets the active, rising primordial energy and a visceral, clear, and nondual awareness dawns in the practitioner.

Psychologically, the awakening of kundalini manifested for me in spontaneous, uproarious laughter at the sheer absurdity of my ordinary mind and in awareness of the intrinsic, pervasive joy that lies behind that realization. Physically, I experienced unusual sounds, sleep disturbance, and a strong vibration, or *spanda*, coursing through my body and said to be a quality of the universal energy. With time, the effects dissipated.

The energy of desire freed from clinging or attachment is key to transformation through this path, something I am still learning. The late Swami Muktananda pointed out that "sexual desire was connected to the process of becoming an *urdhvareta*, from which one gets the power to give Shaktipat. When the svadhisthana chakra is pierced, sexual desire becomes very strong, but this happens so that the flow of sexual fluid may be turned upward" for purposes of gaining liberation or release from worldly attachments.[10] After all, sexual desire is an aspect of the primordial, pure, universal form of desire known as *kama*. According to Tantra, sexual desire is a source of energetic power in the world that can be mastered for higher purposes.

But how can we understand such experiences? According to Silburn, ancient texts explain how

> all along the nadis there are centers, placed one above the other, which the Kundalini has to pierce during her ascent. In ordinary persons these wheels neither revolve nor vibrate, they form inextricable tangles of coils, called accordingly 'knots' (granthi), because they knot spirit and matter, thus strengthening the sense of ego.[11]

She explains the knots near the base of the spine:

> Some of these knots of energy, muladhara and bhru, are not easily loosened. Together they constitute the unconscious complexes (samskara) woven by illusion, and the weight and rigidity of the past offers a strong opposition to the passage of the spiritual force. Each knot, being an obstruction, must be loosened so that the energy released by the centers can be absorbed by Kundalini and thus regain its universality.[12]

These blockages are ultimately caused by the turning of the mind in its relationship to thought, emotion, and the physical body as they interact with life experiences. A corollary experience of kundalini energy is known as *candali* in some Tantric Buddhist texts.

## Intrinsic, Energetic Logic

This upward movement is kundalini's natural and conscious propensity. Therefore, according to Tantra Yoga, it is a built-in human aspiration or desire to seek liberation (*mumukshutva*) from ignorance, attachment, and aggression. That means raising feminine Shakti energy and uniting it with its male Shiva counterpart, supreme wisdom consciousness. Love and compassion, reflected in the open heart, are key prerequisites to the unfolding of this process of transformation. The energetic desire lying within them must be distinguished from our craving and clinging to objects we desire—our hedonism—where a contracted consciousness seeks to desperately envelop and possess objects rather than open to desire's ubiquity.

There can also be a physiological manifestation to this mystifying energetic experience. The same day that my kundalini awakened, I was healed physically in Yoga class. Were the two experiences related? I believe so. In my evening class with Sylvie, I went into full backbend, or *urdhva dhanurasana*, only to experience an auditory crackling in my left palm as it opened and flattened to the ground for the first time in fifteen years. The woman next to me exclaimed, "What was *that*?"

The bones in my palm, including my ring finger, had fused together years earlier. The condition is a genetic disease known as Dupuytren's Contracture, affecting the palm of the hand and fingers, as connective tissue under the skin thickens and shortens, causing contracted cords and nodules to develop in the palm. Consequently, the fingers draw down toward the palm, with the ring and little finger most commonly affected. In my mind, I had always associated that deformed palm with an intense, ill-fated love relationship. Rama Birch, a nationally renowned teacher and founder of Svaroopa Yoga, would tell me at a retreat center a year after my palm flattened that it signified a relationship that was "mis-hand-led." I never forgot the physiologic symbolism, knowing that the energy centers are individually associated with certain behavioral characteristics, body parts, and stages of spiritual growth.

As I stared at my palm in amazement, Sylvie approached me. "Let me see." Studying my now-flattened palm, she shrugged and matter-of-factly said, "This happens sometimes." Mystified by it all, I thanked her. But at the same time, I wasn't sure why I had. These experiences seemed directly related to her, I thought later, a result of her grace (*prasada*).

So what do these experiences mean, and why are they important for us as practitioners? They are not meant to inflate ego or to be worn as badges of accomplishment, nor are they intended to stigmatize those who experience them as mentally imbalanced or deviant. Also, they are not indicative of the liberation or enlightenment of the master who triggers them but of her level of spiritual progress. These experiences embody Paramahansa Yogananda's charge to "seek the unconditioned, indestructible pure Bliss within yourself."[13] Seek the Bliss, not as glorification of the flesh, but to appreciate the good, the beautiful, and the perpetually joyful which is our essential nature as human beings (as opposed to an inherent sinfulness emphasized by some religions). These experiences point toward the more expansive possibilities for healing and insight tied to Yoga as a transformative discipline, to its subtle geography of the body and ethereal storehouse of memory (*smriti*) not recognized by mainstream medicine, and to an inherent body-consciousness.

The healing is a pleasurable rooting-out at a deep level beyond the physical body, yet manifested in it. We find emotional trauma solidified into deformity but released through a liberating elixir. Here, too, is energetic communication between human beings transcending speech and space, where focused attention, will, determination, devotion to a teacher, and compassion for a student trigger a potent energy transmission (*samcara*) that acts as our seeds for metamorphosis. Yet my experiences are but a mere taste of what those dedicated to the Yogic path can know more fully. Without a gifted healer and guide, such experiences are not likely to occur.

These experiences embody the wondrous but wholly pragmatic Yogic worldview, where much more of human experience is first made plausible and then made possible for us to attain. Unfortunately, my experience—a very weak rendition of an *Autobiography of a Yogi*—is countered by so many versions of contorted fitness yogis portrayed in the mass media where deeper experiences are vaguely understood, misrepresented, sensationalized, or neglected altogether.

## Yoga's Everyday Magic

It is easy to juxtapose Yoga as direct apprehension of inner truth through spiritual practice (*pratyaksha*) with the yoga of the superficial—the glitz and hype of a physical approach associated with exercise workouts. Could it be otherwise? Can a competitive electronic media and the American public it seduces grasp Yoga's promise of real transformation without "dumbing it down?" Or would the media trivialize the experience into a tell-all television segment entitled "Esoterica: Yoga's Hidden World?" The segment would be doomed to fail and would only scratch the surface as I have, no doubt placing Yoga in the public mind under the same category of supernatural sensationalism as ghosts, near-death experiences, and UFOs.

Despite yoga's packaged superficiality today, Yoga can manifest as magic in our lives—as an unfolding when we open the body, mind, and heart. There are many teachers across the country who can aid in this process. As Feuerstein cogently notes,

> It is not important whether a teacher can go in and out of mystical states at will, or whether he or she can perform all kinds of paranormal feats or whether he or she can jolt the disciple's nervous system through the transformation of life force. . . . What really matters is whether [one], in effect, works the miracle of spiritual transformation in others.[14]

Obviously, most teachers cannot trigger the deep yet subtle changes in their students that Sylvie can. Such Yoga teachers are a precious few, "wish-fulfilling gems" for those lucky enough to discover them. But many instructors can and do authentically help their students begin to explore themselves as physical, emotional, and spiritual beings.

In this sense, the recent popularizing of yoga provides hope that Yoga's gift to the world can continue to be shared and opened by those who seek its real benefits. Key to this opportunity are the gifted teachers who can point the way as we travel alone while with others on our transformative paths.

CHAPTER SIXTEEN

# Tapas in Taos

We know when we have that special energy and enthusiasm that feels so good we do not want to come down. So we stay up. Soon, Yoga begins to color everything in our lives. It seeps into discussions with store clerks and coworkers, family activities, the things we write about, and the places we visit. It is part love and perhaps a touch of madness—a single-pointed determination to follow a path to its destination. It is tapas, energetic heat and light generated through commitment to Yogic disciplines that purify shariira and create radiance, joy, and happiness. And it can be found today among thousands of practitioners in America's yoga subculture. Classically, tapas is associated with austerities that purify and strengthen us. While it manifests as the white-glow heat of our practice, the real story lies with our motivation: Is it a self-absorbed drive for personal accomplishment, the greater pleasure generated through practice, or the natural movement toward an ever deepening understanding?

For me, having a case of "tapas-itis" means reading all I can about Yoga; asking my teachers to clarify technical issues, and making daily room for asana, pranayama, and meditation. It means living and breathing Yoga, even vacationing in places where I am assured the next hit of that holy heat. With extended time off work, I travel to practice, to discover mountain retreat centers and urban storefront studios, and to meet new friends from across the nation who share my joyful tremors. Admittedly, my motivations are mixed. Some are social and mundane; others are more personal and profound. I am motivated by beautiful places, by the thought of deepening my practice, and by surrounding myself with empathic people who understand this crazy love of mine, since they feel it, too.

## Yoga, Western Style

One trip took me to Taos, New Mexico, where I embraced another Yogic opportunity with enthusiastic zeal. The wild mountain and desert country of northern New Mexico is a perfect place for aficionados to get their next high—where they can unroll that mat, strike that spark, and inhale and exhale slowly. It is a colorful country of contrasts year-round, where squawking black-and-white-winged magpies drown out the melodic songs of the yellow mountain finches, where free-range dogs lord over the ubiquitous adobe bugs with backs of orange-and-black geometric shapes, and where honey-sweetened sopapillas and blue corn bread cut the spicy hot tortilla soup.

Six pueblos of Tewa-speaking people dot the Rio Grande basin, with ancestral villages of the Spanish settlers lying interspersed between mountain and mesa. In May, silver shrubs match aspen, spruce, and juniper greens as the low and high roads from Santa Fe to Taos hug the dry and moist mountainsides, respectively. Yoga is plentiful and diverse in Taos, a town of five thousand permanent residents. This hip arts and ski center north of Santa Fe is imbued with Native culture and with breathtaking scenery of thirteen thousand-foot snowcapped peaks and the deep Rio Grande gorge. Its pueblo has been continuously occupied for over a thousand years.

This place, I surmised at first blush, demanded some adjustments. At seven thousand feet, my fingers swelled slightly, and bottled oxygen was sold to address sleep disorders. Boiling water for tea was also affected by the altitude, and my cup cooled more quickly. This was nothing that this smitten yogi could not handle, I thought.

It is such a treat to find forms of practice that I lack back home. Since there are so many types of yoga today, it takes some sampling to know what fits best with one's level of energy, outlook, and preference. Once I checked into the friendly San Geronimo Lodge, I flipped through the yellow pages to call around for class times. There was fitness yoga at the tennis clubs and spas, Ashtanga at Taos Yoga Center, Kundalini at the Taos Kundalini Yoga and Health Center, *Anusara* at Taos Yoga Rhythms, and restorative yoga at Prana Yoga. For my time in Taos, I chose four days of Anusara, having had an initial taste from a class with Texan John Friend, its founder, at a mountain retreat in 2000.

## A Long and Winding Road

I stopped for directions at the World Cup Expresso Caffé in downtown Taos, where the mountaineering and ski crowd meet alternative artists, as environmental activists chat with cowboys and city tourists. T-shirts sold inside begged the java crowd to "resist mediocrity." That should be easy enough, I thought, in a place where Julia Roberts and Donald Rumsfeld own homes, where Pretty Woman lives with the Bomber of Baghdad.

Yoga Rhythms, the Anusara studio, is five miles north of downtown, nestled in a small set of shops sharing a long wooden porch. I pulled into the parking lot and entered the studio through the sliding front door. I was surprised to see the class already in session. A woman to my left in *swastikasana,* a seated pose, asked me to go back out and re-enter around the back, where I would find a blanket and block. She met me there, and we entered the practice space together.

Victoria Carroccio, the owner and sole teacher, is a slender, thirty-something dynamo with long, ponytailed brown hair. More commonly known as Amani, she is formally trained in Yoga teaching at Kripalu and in Anusara by John Friend. She also has had training in Feldenkrais, pilates, and massage therapy. Her quick laughter, good-natured teasing, and articulate micro-movement instructions make it easy to enter her world of shoulder loops and kidney lifts. In her class, I tried to keep up in unfamiliar variations of familiar poses.

My mornings were spent doing Anusara in sunny sixty-five-degree weather, preceded by student chatter of skiing the six-inch snowfall on Kachina Peak. Even in yoga class, I soon realized, one found the contrasts that so readily marked this place. As the days passed, I learned a new yoga lexicon as rich and colorful as this land, while challenging the mediocrity of my personal practice: "Now slide into down dog, spreading your legs further apart, bending your left foot and placing your straightened right behind it, twisting open to the sky." "In the shoulder loop, find the balance of structure and freedom." Afterward, my body felt simultaneously achy and energized.

Anusara, literally "flowing grace" or "following the heart," is much like that slow, winding, and majestic high road from Santa Fe to Taos. Most take the faster and smoother low road, a flowing highway like the common yoga style, vinyasa. But the high road is grand and challenging to traverse, with its multiple bendy switchbacks. Since 1997, John Friend and some of his main teachers—Desiree Rumbaugh, Amy Ippoliti, and Todd Norian among them—have shared his heart-based system of Hatha Yoga to focus upon "universal principles of alignment" informed by the nondual Tantric philosophy taught by Gurumayi. In this Yoga style, mind and body are sacred containers for the expression of supreme consciousness as primordial energy, opening the tender heart to the present moment without clinging or control. That means practitioners are "freed to be in the flow," as students are asked and sometimes challenged to recognize their basic goodness despite feelings they have or judgments they make to the contrary.

## Yoga Discipline as an Art Form

Amani did not teach classes on the weekend, so this Yoga madman scored his next hit elsewhere. Arroyo Seco is a tiny hamlet of tourist shops on the road to the Taos Ski Valley. Cloaked in fluttering Tibetan prayer flags, the entrance to Prana Yoga Studio is directly behind a colorful shop of hand-painted pillows and T-shirts with splashes of yellows, golds, reds, and greens. I sat on the wooden porch bench waiting for the teacher and students to arrive for the 11 a.m. restorative class.

Staring up at the snowcapped mountains with a clear blue sky background, I reflected on how, like Taos, I was full of such glaring contrasts—serious and thoughtful at one moment, silly and absurd at the next; how my unquestioned commitment and determination to keep up my practice were fed partly by the way I felt in my body, just like a drug addict; and how like an addictive substance, Yoga's practices transformed me physically and psychologically, gradually and dramatically, and yet my fix was more than its outcome. It was the joy of having an amorphous, diffuse community of teachers and practitioners—my ability to travel fourteen hundred miles from home and find that Amani, previously a stranger, knew the same challenges, feelings of accomplishment and humility, and Yoga teachers in Massachusetts. I was part of a much larger subculture, I concluded, and that further reinforced my commitment.

But it was also more than that. After the Saturday Prana class, I drove back toward town, stopping at Taos Tin Works, where I struck up a conversation with Marion Moore, who has been in business for more than fifteen years. "What brings you here?" Marion asked. "Yoga. I'm here to practice, to write, and to enjoy what the area has to offer." She told me that she had done yoga over the years but had never been able to stick with it. "So what keeps you so committed?" she wondered. I answered, "I think it takes a lot of determination at first, and you begin to feel so good, so accomplished, so enthusiastic for more. Later, as you do more practices, you ride on that energy, that love, which carries you to go even deeper. And as you dive deeper, you confront and move right through the fears, the knots, the impediments that previously had held you back in class and in life. And you feel so free." Marion gave me a curious smile and a nod of the head. "Just like my art."

Climbing back into my car, I realized that a particular type of love fueled my "tapas-itis," neither a desperate manic fixation nor an unhealthy attachment. It is the broad love that John Friend talks about—feeling fully alive in the body and having a zest for life—that carries me out into the world, to this place, and simultaneously back into my mind and body. Perhaps more precisely, it is the feeling of tenderness and appreciation for both the journey and goal that my Yoga offers. In the purest sense, whenever the duality falls away, Yoga *is* that very zest for living life fully, that sweet sense of well-being—sukkha—where the aim and motivation of Yoga remain clear without clinging to the pleasurable sensations of my practice. In those fleeting moments of nondual awareness, Yoga becomes our experience of life, and we become Yoga.

As the sun set on the bendy Rio Grande, I looked out the window on my return flight and silently reviewed my Taos experience. From such distance, I more easily saw how that ancient and contemporary gemstone below me held a special place in my personal history of Yoga practice. It was where I looked into Yoga's reflection—a wild, contrasting, yet perfect tapestry—and found that I myself was the madness which should not be overcome, lest I lose the spark which kept me feeding the wellspring that is my practice, that is my life.

## CHAPTER SEVENTEEN

# EMILY'S HEART

Leafing through yoga magazines gives the reader a good idea of the retreat options available today on the yoga marketplace. There is Hatha instruction in a lush Costa Rican rainforest, hobnobbing with yoga celebrities on a Caribbean cruise, and a rest and relaxation weekend at a mountain retreat center. They hardly begin to scratch the surface of the options available today.[1] While many retreats offer "fun in the sun," other getaways provide a safe haven for a healing process to unfold, where those suffering from life situations that create pain or sorrow can take the initiative to tend to themselves and where mundane concerns like fixing meals or structuring one's day are handled by others. Either saying nothing or sharing are equally respected, and attendees can feel free to "just be." As a result, mood swings, feelings of anger, or sadness are fully recognized and honored as part of the healing process.

## APPLYING AHIMSA

On a Yoga retreat a few years ago, I met Emily, a woman who applied ahimsa, or nonharming, in her own life in such a courageous way that her heart opened despite years of enduring intense emotional pain. Ahimsa is the supreme yama, or behavioral restraint, of the Yogic path, and it is central to Indian spiritual philosophies. It relates to how we treat others as well as ourselves. When ahimsa comes into apparent conflict with other yamas, it trumps them. In extreme cases, even *satya*, or truth-telling, is secondary to protecting others from harm.

A pretty, petite seventy-year-old housewife, Emily had decided to increase her knowledge of Yoga philosophy, the asanas, and breath work. Talkative and timid, she wore a gentle, sad smile. Upon meeting me, she confided her nervousness over the lack of locked doors at the mountain retreat, where a quarter of the visitors were men. When our class turned to a discussion of satya, she shared a story that had remained foremost in her mind.

Emily's father had been a physician, and her family lived on a large estate bordering tall woodlands. On a beautiful autumn evening, her father had finished his rounds at a local Connecticut hospital and asked his daughter to join him after dinner for a walk as her mother did the dishes. Emily adored this tall, middle-aged man and took advantage of any chance to spend time with him. She recalled the warm breeze on her face, the smell of dampness, and the swishing sound as they shuffled through piles of golden leaves. She would remember this day every day for fifty-five years. As dusk settled on the thick forest, Emily's father grabbed her, forced himself on her, and raped her. She would never forget the smell, the taste, the touch, and the heartbreak of that day. A sheltering silence between them would mark their relationship for years.

The nearly lifelong legacy of a now-dead father could be found in Emily's body and mind, in the fear of unlocked places where strange men were present, in apprehension over an unprotected granddaughter alone with a son-in-law, and in the timidity and nervousness with which she spoke of these things. But now she felt intuitively that Yoga would help her accept and more fully integrate this life experience and would help reveal the truth in healing from her life trauma.

Elisabeth Kübler-Ross and David Kessler, in *On Grief and Grieving*, note how engaging with the grief process is fundamental to healing, moving us from deadened to vital while acknowledging the devastation that has come before. Some sexual assault treatment programs operate loosely on the basis of Kübler-Ross's well-known paradigm of healing from life crises: denial, anger, depression, bargaining, and acceptance.[2] Before entering our Yoga retreat, Emily felt that she had learned through therapy to stay with the healing process by acknowledging her anger and depression. Now, she had begun to focus her continuing recovery on a growing commitment to Yoga and to a breath work that kept her focused in the body through movement. She learned to breathe into the physical and emotional trauma while exhaling it out. Now, she had begun to refocus her meditative practice on the suffering of others, breathing in their pain while breathing out love and light.

## A Healing Worldview

Kübler-Ross and Kessler stress the need for a new worldview in working with a healing process like Emily's: "Your belief system needs to heal and regroup as much as your soul does. You must start to rebuild a belief system from the foundation up, one that has room for the realities of life and still offers safety and hope for a different life: a belief system that will ultimately have a beauty of its own to be discovered with life and loss."[3] For Emily, this belief system involved Eastern philosophies—including Hinduism, Taoism, and Buddhism—and the promise Yoga and meditation held for personal transformation, for *her* transformation.

Indian philosophies—including the six darshanas, or views, in Hinduism and the major schools of Buddhism—can appear daunting at times, even when explaining suffering and its relationship to the human predicament. Yet they also offer practical worldviews for addressing our life experiences—both in understanding why tragedies occur and how we might work with them—while providing pragmatic means for addressing our thoughts, feelings, and actions. By helping us to acknowledge our present situations and to "see things as they are," these philosophies lay a foundation for consciously working with the mind and body in gaining acceptance of all that has ever happened to us. By stabilizing the reflective mind—that source of so much of our ongoing dissatisfaction through self-judgment—we begin to realize that we are fine just the way we are. By working with life-force energy through Yoga postures and breath work, we see more clearly how we are obstructed from feeling whole again. Honest exploration of thoughts and feelings as they arise from moment to moment is the basis for our healing, slowly but directly, regardless of the trauma that we might confront.

This is never an easy process, especially when dealing with the aftermath of rape by a loved one. But while acknowledging and sharing her feelings, Emily had arrived at acceptance of her past and of her father—no longer seeing him as the devil; no longer blaming herself; and no longer feeling frozen, impotent, and absorbed in her pain. The occasional panic attacks, flashbacks, and felt disengagement from her body waned with time. For Emily, the legacy of her father could now be found in her heart. Despite any mixed emotions or confused feelings, as Emily tells it, she loved him to his dying day. *She loves him to this day.* This brought tears to the eyes of retreat participants as we listened in silence and support. Afterward, Emily hugged me and wore the broad, sweet smile of personal accomplishment.

Later, I wondered if I could cultivate such a wide open heart, an Emily's heart, to love someone who had victimized *me*, who had so hurt me to leave an inheritance of fear and sadness and shame, an inheritance that could dissolve like water into air under the emotional intensity of a loving community. Now, I occasionally retell Emily's story in my Yoga classes, because I have found that it also liberates me. The heart is a truly spiritual organ of transformation that knows no limits except for those imposed by the mind. Emily's story makes me feel that I can broaden my heart. It provides me with a gentle touchstone if I feel my heart begin to harden throughout the day. That is Emily's personal legacy for me.

## The Heart Connection

Laureen Smith practices yoga therapy with sexual abuse survivors. She explains how such trauma creates emotional blockages and impairs personal growth and healing at the various energy centers of the body. At anahata, or the heart chakra, for example, she notes that

> the love, spaciousness, and open quality of the air element of this chakra can be "sucked dry," especially when the perpetrator of abuse was someone the survivor trusted. Love of oneself, love of life, love (and trust) of another are all compromised by abuse. Asanas that both soften the heart and open the chest can bring sensation and balance back to this area. Backbends are particularly powerful for healing of this chakra, as is ujayi pranayama. . . . Learning to open the heart and expand the rib cage—connecting the lower chakras with the upper—becomes the yogic challenge of this area.[4]

This was the challenge that Emily had met and integrated with her life situation after so many years.

In *The Places That Scare You*, Buddhist nun Pema Chödrön notes that "forgiveness . . . cannot be forced. When we are brave enough to open our hearts to ourselves, however, forgiveness will emerge."[5] Emily opened her heart to herself by publicly exposing an ancient wound to fresh air and feeling the prickly warmth of healing toward the one who had wielded the blade. Committing to Yoga and finding a container safe for expressing deep feelings served as the perfect incubation for Emily's continued growth in courage and forgiveness. A sense of freedom and exhilaration seems to naturally arise as we escape so many years of wearing the heavy, suffocating armor of our secret lives.

Perhaps a universal quality of being human is confronting such feelings of victimization, no matter how small, through incidents of verbal, emotional, or physical abuse. After all, we meet with aggressive responses all the time—the casual shove out of frustration; the "Oh, shut up" when disapproving of another; and reflexive anger when cut off in traffic. Emily's lesson teaches us that we can find the strength to heal from even the most heinous forms of aggression by letting go—dropping the role of victim by recognizing, accepting, and sharing our love and ending the victim-victimizer dance.

Pema Chödrön offers us the blueprint for such transformations in the form of specific meditations that open the heart. "First we acknowledge what we feel—shame, revenge, embarrassment, remorse. Then we forgive ourselves for being human. Then, in the spirit of not wallowing in the pain, we let go and make a fresh start." She concludes, "We will discover forgiveness as a natural expression of the open heart."[6]

This is the challenge for followers of Yoga's transformative pathway—to apply the yamas, or behavioral restraints, to our lives in a direct and visceral way. Through Emily's experience, we see how the virtue of ahimsa demands from us intuitive wisdom, knowing that suffering will occur if we coerce, manipulate, and hurt others through our bodies, speech, or minds. Ahimsa also requires compassion, absolving those who harm us and forgiving ourselves if we had neither the strength nor the wisdom to have done anything about it.

CHAPTER EIGHTEEN

18

# Indra's Net

*All human events are rooted in*
*the law of cause and effect. . . .*
*In this life, you are the architect of your own destiny.*
—Paramahansa Yogananda

Even logical, analytical, and data-driven people can be open to life's inexplicable mysteries. A skeptical, number-crunching administrator in my professional life, just show me the facts and that is all I need. So when I have told my story to colleagues and acquaintances, some seem more than a little perplexed but perhaps not totally surprised. After all, I am happily married with a healthy commitment to Yoga and meditation, which together feed my perspective, priorities, and private life.

For two decades, I have been a client of a gifted psychic who is a nonresidential member of the Ananda Community, which follows the teachings of Swami Paramahansa Yogananda and Swami Kriyananda. A blond-haired, level-headed, and street-savvy woman in her fifties, Kathryn Kendall reads Tarot cards in Portland, Oregon, and provides me with tapes of her predictions. While researching the New Age in the 1980s, I initially thought that a stranger forecasting my future using cards of Asian origin, with images drawn from the European Renaissance, would be highly inaccurate. But over the years, she would accurately predict my relationship with my wife, job offers, crises, house purchases, home construction, my mother's serious injury and death, and even the publication of this book. As a clairvoyant, Kathryn sees her clients as living, breathing mirrors with future knowledge reflected back through the subtle symbolism of the cards, or through their "sacred geometry of chance," as the rock star Sting once sang.

A few years ago, Kathryn stunned me.

> Through your Yoga life, you're going to get closer to a young person. You're fifty, and maybe they're twenty-eight or thirty. At first, you're going to think, 'What do I have in common with this person?' But the more you talk, the more it will feel like slipping into an old pair of comfy Levis. It will feel so right. But please don't scare them. You see, you knew each other in the past, and you were so happy together. Don't freak them out. They probably don't understand about past lives.

Past lives? Kathryn had never mentioned anything about my past before—my *really* distant past. While reincarnation is often treated with romantic sentimentality in movies and plain goofiness on the cultural fringe, it is a tangible reality in Yoga. Our personal, social, and physical identities are products of this life and will not survive death. But they are also manifestations of our actions in a previous life. Depending on the tradition, the soul or subtle consciousness is said to pass from one body to another, transmitting karmic seeds or propensities accumulated through our lifetimes. The *kleshas*, or mental states, from which these seeds of reaction sprout are the momentum, or force, of rebirth. Every sense-experience and thought (vritti) form samskaras, or subtle reactive imprints on the mind, that are potentially transmitted into the future. Training the mind to change one's samskaras is a potential outcome of serious Yoga practice. I knew Kathryn could read my future—perhaps a result of some unique connection between us—but could she see my past as well?

## TOUCHING HIGHER CONSCIOUSNESS

Noted Jungian psychotherapist Marie-Louise von Franz points out, in *On Divination and Synchronicity*, that the universal Energy-Consciousness she calls the unconscious, "knows things: it knows the past and future, it knows things about other people. . . . A medium is a person who has a closer relationship, one might say a gift, by which to relate to the absolute knowledge of the unconscious"—a gift to see the meaning in the chaotic mosaic of geometric relationships laid out in the cards before her.[1] Kathryn continued: "This is not a love affair, Tom. It is deep friendship with love involved. So I have a warning for you. Don't get attached. This is not a time for the two of you to be together. Love them, but let them go."

Those who have clairvoyance, known as a *siddhi* or spiritual power to Yogis, have access to our future thoughts and feelings, even if we do not give them permission to unlock such secrets. Gifted practitioners on the Yogic path are called siddha yogis (which, by her own admission, Kathryn is not), and they are capable of performing incredible feats as a natural by-product of their advancement. Those of us lucky enough to benefit from such predictions are obliged to treat such hidden knowledge with care. Over time, I had come to view Kathryn's readings as both a blessing and a curse, warning and comforting me about near-disasters while eliciting hope and fear that pulled me out of the present moment and into an occasional cycle of worry and wishful thinking. Yet I would not obsess about her predictions if they seemed far-fetched, highly improbable, or of little interest to me.

Months passed, and I had forgotten about Kathryn's prophecy. I returned home from attending a medical conference in Midtown

Manhattan. Entering my teacher's evening yoga class, I introduced myself to Ginny, an attractive young woman who had relocated from out of state. This introduction was nothing out of the ordinary for me, I thought. But this *felt* different. So fascinated and so at ease in talking to her, I asked this single, unattached fellow student out for tea.

"What's wrong with me?" I wondered to myself afterward as if drawn by an unavoidable magnetic energy with mounting desire and attraction to Ginny. I recited a mantra-like affirmation over and over again in my mind: "I am happy. I feel so alive. I have a devoted, loving mate. Is this what midlife crises are like? Why am I so drawn to this woman?"

The easy answer would be that the situation amounted to a self-fulfilling prophecy, that I was predisposed to find someone since I was told to expect them, or that I unconsciously longed for such a relationship. But there had to be more to it. After all, I reasoned, you cannot just make these things happen, and I was not consciously looking for anyone. Or was I? Was this strong attraction my "Lost-in-Translation" midlife trauma driven by biology, shortened years, and a receding hairline?

My experience with Kathryn's predictions is that I cannot easily or deliberately stop events from happening, regardless of the reasons for their appearance. Why should this situation be any different, I thought? An accurate prediction did not mean my life was preordained, only that my actions had conditions and consequences that could not be easily foreseen but that could be forecasted by the gifted. Von Franz writes that "in different techniques of divination one sees that actual events are never predicted, but only the quality of possible events. . . . The prediction only refers to the quality of the moment in which a synchronistic event might occur."[2] And in my experience with Kathryn, it is also the case that some predictions do not reflect this quality of the moment so that there is often some ambiguity. They prompt me to think about the decisions I make, which is their great value to me.

As Ginny and I got to know each other over a period of months, I recognized our similarities, despite differences in age, experience, beauty, and temperament. We were both looking for new jobs; we had a penchant for reflecting on our feelings; felt an emotional distance from extended families; had similar professional ambitions; and shared a love of practice. Such mundane similarities are not uncommon among confidants. But I felt an uncanny synchronicity from the very beginning—meaningful coincidences; an ease to our intimate conversations; identical statements spoken at the very same moment; the same motivations for previous marriages; a feeling of immediate camaraderie; and an awareness of a lurking danger behind our budding friendship.

Intuitively, I knew Ginny and I shared that same unspoken understanding. Yet I felt so intensely drawn to her, such a strong pull of attachment (raga) that it scared me. Yes, we would need to end our conversations of emotional intimacy and physical innocence and we slowly pulled away, hesitantly and unevenly at first, awkwardly at best. This pulling away was emotionally difficult for me, as I continued to see her occasionally in class. Yet Kathryn's words of advice echoed in my mind. *Love her*, but let her go. Love her, but *let her go*. We let our unlikely friendship go.

As von Franz suggests, "for everything there is a right moment, the right constellation for action and to act too early or too late destroys the whole possibility."[3] Kathryn has made accurate predictions since but none with the same emotional investment for me. A primal sadness lingered for some time, and I wondered why this smart, ambitious, and headstrong young woman stood out as so special among the hundreds of people I would meet each year around the country.

I turned to the Yogic path, my anchor and compass, for guidance—meditating to watch my fluctuating thoughts, journaling to explore my feelings without judgment, confiding in an empathic power yoga teacher to gain perspective, and meeting with a psychologist who shared my Yogic sensibilities to uncover a deeper understanding of my circumstance. Each step allowed me to more fully embrace the situation while loosening my attachment to see things more clearly.

## Karmic Dance

As our lives move through time, like spacecraft circling the earth, the horizon of possible events rotates before us and eventually comes into full view. As a psychic, Kathryn places chance at the very center of her readings to predict the likelihood of meaningful coincidences occurring beyond the visible horizon of possibility. From her perspective, events take place for a higher, broader purpose tied to our spiritual development. Our karma—the positive or negative consequences of previous actions—has meaning that often transcends our ability to understand it fully or rationally at the moment actions or their consequences occur.

Before engaging in regular meditation practice, I used to assume that life events were largely random, chance occurrences to which I assigned meaning and importance. Like an armchair scientist, I would informally compute the probability that certain events would occur as long as I could identify, control, and manipulate the assumed causes, eliminating chance to try to bring about a desired end—love, happiness, or career success. My control usually did not work. As my relationship with Kathryn deepened over time and, aided by practice and self-study, my shallow understanding gave way to trusting life's natural flow and deeper meaning.

This act of surrendering my ego-personality's sense of attachment and control is symbolized by commitment to the niyama of *Ishwara-Pranidhana*. Ishwara represents the embodiment of the Absolute and of limitless wisdom, and our devotion to it results from our surrender, effort, and intuitive understanding. While our ego-mind tells us to maintain a firm grip on situations that seem to be falling out of our control, Yoga philosophy teaches that through such a grip we can create knots in our bodies that block the flow of energy. If we learn to listen to our higher self—our intuitive wisdom—we recognize that it is natural to let go (*vairagya*).

## Growth Opportunity

One Saturday morning, I ran into my old friend, Linda, at a lakeshore coffee shop. In the course of catching up with each other's lives, our conversation gravitated to my earlier experience. "Ever see that Ginny you once told me about?" she asked pointedly.

"No, not really. I have had time and emotional distance to integrate that experience, to put it into context, maybe a higher context."

We seem to have a lower and higher self—that ego-clinging self, grasping at pleasures and desires, and an all-knowing, higher consciousness which we tap into when we settle the reflective mind and allow our innate wisdom to unfold. The energy generated through Yoga has to be acknowledged and respected. As I felt more fully alive through practice, I realized that I had a responsibility to acknowledge desire as it arises and channel its energy into ways that are appropriate, given my commitments, like a brahmacharyan who carefully nurtures his energy.

I lowered my voice. "I have thought a lot about that experience. My feelings of tenderness and affection for people are authentic; they're real, but that doesn't mean they are harbingers of any specific outcome. You know the old 'soul-mate syndrome' that some people fall into. Through Yoga, I have learned to spread my wings outward from my heart toward many people. My challenge is not to let my desire 'get stuck' on any one person but to keep opening to the world around me. I think that is the essence of Yoga as a spiritual path." I paused to choose my words carefully. "Only with Ginny, it felt so special, so intense. I had totally lost my equanimity. I'm afraid that any special energetic connection with someone doesn't guarantee anything in an absolute sense. Perhaps all I wanted, all

I desired, was to affirm what we saw in each other—someone worthy of being loved unconditionally."

Harvard-trained psychiatrist Mark Epstein draws on the Tantric tradition to explain the role of desire in our personal transformations: "Allowing ourselves into desire's abyss turns out to be the key to a more complete enjoyment of its fruits. By experiencing desire in its totality: gratifying and frustrating; sweet and bitter; pleasant and painful; successful and yet coming up short, we can use it to awaken our minds."[4] In other words, turning away from desire is never the answer if we wish to live fully and happily. Intense desire can both fuel our search for release from suffering and enslave us through attachment to objects. The key lies in "forsaking the acting out that clinging creates"[5] while recognizing any emotional confusion (*sammoha*) that disrupts the serenity of our minds and senses of purpose. If the term "soul mate" has a deeper meaning, as author Elizabeth Gilbert once pondered, might it refer to those people entering our lives who transform us through the energetic power of desire?

Love, desire, tenderness, and compassion are intrinsic to living fully. Yoga teaches us that obsessive attachment to objects—the clinging—will not bring lasting happiness, only great psychological suffering. *Mohan* (temptation or infatuation) is the resulting delusion, overlooking any negatives of the object or situation to which we grow attached. On a mundane level, emotionally intense experiences like mine can be reduced to playing out a childhood drama, responding to an earlier unresolved event, or simply following an old relationship script brought to the surface until we learn to see it for what it is, finally handling it artfully and compassionately. "You know, maybe I'm like that Hanged Man in the Tarot deck," I surmised. "Really hung up until I got it right. When pursuing intimacy and affirmation as a young man, all too often I was snared by the clinging that my desire generated."

Kathryn may have been accurate in predicting my past, but that did not mean her interpretations were always on the money. "Other than a handful of highly evolved beings, who really knows about our past lives? I don't. I prefer to think fondly on the whole situation now," I concluded. "A brief, intense interlude in my happily married life; a profound mutual test; a feeling of immediate tenderness and affection for someone; and a reminder of life's potent possibilities, of choices made and honored, of potential karmic consequences foreseen," and of the yama *asteya*—not taking what we desire that does not belong to us.

"Maybe Joseph Campbell was right about human love," Linda responded, alluding to that great scholar of human mythology.[6] "One can have what he called a 'love seizure' even if you're married. These are precious moments, and they don't happen often in our lives. If you don't respond to it, it dulls the whole vitality of love, the whole freefall of pure desire."

I nodded and smiled: "Maybe, but it felt so dangerous, so threatening to all that I find comfortable and stable and important, all that I have built up—the edifice of my life." And maybe that is the point. All that we build as architects of our own destinies is impermanent and can come tumbling down at a moment's notice, through our own and others' volition.

As we hugged goodbye, I realized that I had come to terms with an emotionally intense event that seemed so natural and special and yet equally absorbing and troubling. I had descended into an old habitual pattern of grasping and attachment to something only apparently real and concrete, and I was unable to acknowledge the pleasurable energy without getting stuck on the object of desire. Only by not pushing these situations away are we able to address and even overcome unconscious complexes woven by illusion as part of our processes of transformation. This challenge at finding peace is not unlike ones we all face at some point, caught as we are in Indra's Net—that great web of karmic interactions.

And as we stabilize and focus our minds through Yoga, we may not be able to foresee future probabilities as siddha yogis or as Kathyrn can. But we may be able to clearly see that auspicious coincidences are indeed natural and that their magic permeates everything around us, including those we encounter in a Yoga class. Our challenge is to recognize this simple yet wondrous truth as part of our lives, this great Yogic experiment in living.

## CHAPTER NINETEEN

# Poison and Antidote

The body of the nineteen-year-old woman, hands tied behind her back, was found face down on his Wiltshire estate. Ritually murdered, she would come to symbolize the life of this world-famous yogi, this agnostic who had proclaimed in song that "there is no religion but sex and music."

Cosmopolitan in reach, eclectic in style, and ever-evolving in sight and sound, Gordon Sumner, better known as Sting, has been called the thinking person's songwriter. His lyrics borrow from Greek mythology, English history, his personal sorrows and loves lost, political realities, and fictional characters trapped by circumstance and choice. His recognizable sound owes to the heritage of world music, and his words occasionally to the legacy of a five thousand-year-old Yogic worldview.

Regularly practicing Ashtanga, Sting is among the most famous yogis of the international community. In 1993, he did a series of asanas on the music video for his international tour, *Ten Summoner's Tales*. By the time the yoga explosion hit America, Sting appeared in full shoulder stand on the cover of his CD, *Brand New Day*, and had harmonized on kirtan master Krishna Das's CD, *Pilgrim Heart*.

And *Yoga Journal* reported in June of 2001 that Sting had taught an asana class to contest winners in Los Angeles, the perfect setting for someone who had once sung that "Every breath you take, every move you make, I'll be watching you." But who has been watching *him*?

It seems that everybody has—from millennium revelers and Super Bowl fans to audiences at his knighting as a Citizen of the British Empire and at the 2007 Grammy Awards. That the young and middle-aged alike are drawn to packed arenas and tours on six continents attests to Sting's sustained appeal. His 2004 "*Sacred Love*" tour was second highest in box office gross sales in North America,[1] and his autobiography *Broken Music* helps us understand the man behind the celebrity mask, taking us to his doorstep of stardom with The Police. It is a story of unsettled alienation and discontent—of dukkha—and a long-sought peace.

## Life as Unsatisfactory

Yoga teaches us that we create our destinies moment by moment. Therefore, we are ultimately responsible for our happiness as well as our dissatisfaction. Gordon Sumner understands this. Born of northern England's urban working class, Sumner's insecurities from a confused childhood evolved into the struggles of an angry and driven youth who attended university and taught school in the 1970s while moonlighting as a jazz musician. His ambition masked an inner turmoil and dissatisfaction. "I think my life has progressed from being a very unhappy child," he would tell the *Sunday Independent*.[2]

According to Yogic philosophy, dukkha, or life's unsatisfactory quality, results from not seeing things clearly and is tied to obstacles known as the "three poisons"—ignorance, attachment or greed, and aggression.[3] First, we do not see our true nature or True Self clearly. Rather, we strongly associate with our physical body and ego-personality, searching for pleasure and avoiding pain. We cling to pleasurable sensory objects and evade their opposites—whether as people, places, things, or experiences. This clinging often solidifies through our judgments and opinions, evolving into a source of frustration or discontent. We oscillate between the Scylla of hope and the Charybdis of fear. Frustrated at not being able to control what we desire, we feel anger and soon we externalize the issue at hand by blaming others. Or we escape through avoidance or melancholy, an aggression turned inward. Without insight, we repeat this cycle for a lifetime.

The three poisons are the cause of our suffering. Peace, or release from their entanglement, comes from regular practice of Yoga, including meditation, and through serious self-study. The three poisons are universal, challenging even those whom we think have everything—wealth, fame, beauty, brains, and power—including Sting.

## THE BOOK OF HIS LIFE

Sting's early life was off center; he was a stranger growing up in his own home: "I felt like I was in the wrong place," he admitted in that *Sunday Independent* interview. He loved his parents, but his father was emotionally distant, and his mother loved another man throughout his childhood. Gordon would catch them in each other's arms. The resulting confusion, frustration, and anger, he admits, haunted his later relationships with women, and he eventually refused to attend either of his parents' funerals: "Escape and the need to keep moving had by now become endemic in me."

His challenges included early marriage, young fatherhood, and the ethical dilemma and emotional trauma caused by unfaithfulness and divorce. While not proud of the domestic mess of that time, he had fallen madly in love with his present wife, actress and film producer Trudie Styler. "That I have managed to maintain even a modicum of my sanity through this period is owed more to Trudie's love, and patient faith in my deeper self," he wrote in his autobiography.[4] First married in 1992, Gordon and Trudie have remained happy together for more than twenty years and have four children and seven homes on two continents.

Sting's self-admitted workaholism has yielded fortune, unimagined fame almost unparalleled among British pop stars, and an uncanny four-decade evolution in both thought and style. But it also demands frequent separation from Trudie and the children. Perhaps a key to Sting's creativity is this dance between connection, disconnection, and reconnection. "You have to allow yourselves to evolve," or as he explained in song: "If you love somebody, set them free." His commitment includes a respect for the role of separation in intimacy.

Sting's musical themes suggest a complicated man, emerging from the simple, raw driving rock beat and sad sexual desperation of "Roxanne" to the sophisticated Indian instrumentation and nuanced lyrics of love and reincarnation in "A Thousand Years." "My personal life is in my songs, in an archetypal form," he noted on his Web site. "To a certain extent, my songs are abstract, but if I look at them closely I can see that I'm writing about my private life," a life that has evolved to find greater love and acceptance through his composing, his self-reflection, and his Yoga practice.

Sting's songwriting spans a wide swath of human situations and a depth of complexity that reflect a fertile imagination—a transvestite street prostitute asking for neither acceptance nor condemnation; a hot-wiring car thief imagining the compromised life of his wealthy victim; a pirate's bride waiting for her dead sweetheart to return from the other side of the world; and a laid-back suitor given an ultimatum, a demand for an answer in seven days. The examples jump off the music sheet—predicaments begging for resolution, for freedom from stress, isolation, deprivation, and heartbreak. They are lives slightly off-kilter or conditions undeserved. "I think I've only written one song. It's about feeling trapped and gaining release," he told a reporter from the *Daily Telegraph*.[5]

This, too, is the story of his Yoga practice—feeling constricted, listening to inner wisdom, and loosening the grip. By 1991, Danny Paradise had introduced Sting to yoga, and he soon began daily practice of ashtanga vinyasa, among other forms. Through a seventeen-year commitment, Sting has worked to cultivate synchrony of mind and body: "It's about control and letting go, compulsion and release. Being goal-oriented but also having to surrender," he explained in that same interview. The psychological process central to Yoga practice, coupled with his keen self-examination, allowed Sting to closely examine the workings of his mind—how he handled situations and caused rancor or ill feeling. This process seemed to manifest in his transformation as an artist and performer as well as in priorities he gave to his physical surroundings. He created a garden labyrinth on his estate that helps calm and clear his mind.[6]

Sting explained the physical, psychological, and spiritual benefits of Yoga to *Yoga Journal* five years after first practicing:

> When I really do my Yoga in the morning, I have more energy in the day. I get more done. My mind is more composed. There are more benefits to it than I would have thought. They are not just physical, but mental and I am even coming to believe that they are spiritual. . . . The deeper you get into Yoga you realize, yes, it is a spiritual practice. . . . It's not the first reason I did it. But I suppose that as I get older and I get more contemplative, the Yoga practice will take that on. Especially the breathing, which is linked very closely to meditation.[7]

## Inner and Outer Transformation

The creative force behind The Police spread his solo wings to become a Grammy Award-winning artist by the early 1990s. This period, just before his foray into the fusion of international sounds, marks Sting's transition to a more centered and satisfied person. By the 1993 release of *Ten Summoner's Tales*, the king of pain had learned to walk in fields of gold. Overcoming the inner demons of his early career, Sting admitted on a PBS special covering his tour that "I don't have to be going through a trauma or spiritual negativity to make a record. I can virtually be happy and content to write songs that are essentially amusing."

And he did write amusing songs. He talked to the devil in hell, given his mystical attraction to his best friend's woman. He promised to wash himself more often to please a perpetually dissatisfied girlfriend. Facing a six-foot-ten Neanderthal rival, he described himself as the Mighty Flea. Despite the press's claims of pretension, Sting has never been afraid to expose his vulnerability.

His contemplative nature and curiosity have been evident throughout his career and more so as he has become more comfortable with himself. Struggle with inner demons in his early career gives way to synthesized resolutions of diverse international sounds—whimsically Caribbean on *The Living Sea* CD*;* Indo-Arabic stylization and French hip-hop on *Brand New Day;* techno, blues, and jazz beat on *Sacred Love* (which also includes the sitar maestro Anoushka Shankar); and more recently, Renaissance music for lute on *Songs from the Labyrinth.* At times, his lyrics are embedded with universal symbols of our earthiness: birth, desire, energy, destruction, and regeneration. He is a man sensitive to the natural cycles and needs of the earth—an organic gardener and co-founder of the Rainforest Foundation—and to those of humankind—a proponent of Amnesty International and of nuclear disarmament. It is not surprising that he was honored as MusiCares Person of the Year in 2003.

Sting was brought up Catholic, but he lost his faith in the holy church. Science and progress would fare no better. From an early age, music became his blessed sacrament. "Music is the one spiritual force in our lives that we still have access to. . . . It saved my sanity," he admitted on his 1993 tour. Often reduced to an interest in esoteric sexuality, his Tantra practice is "about reconnecting with the world of the spirit through everyday things," as he explained in the *Sunday Independent* interview. Often asked about Tantra's sexual overtones by journalists seeking sensationalism, he merely replies, "The tantric aim is to ritualize sex more, and not be so perfunctory." The so-called "left-hand Tantric schools" focus on ritualized, extended sexual union as an avenue for spiritual liberation that some today mistake for a hedonistic hyper-ecstasy. Sting has been known to quip that four-hour sessions with his wife include an hour of begging and pleading as well as a dinner and movie.

How does Sting feel about God? He again sings the Tantric tune of a universal, primordial energy. "He-she-it doesn't look like you and he doesn't look like me. . . . It's surely an inclusive concept, it includes everything, the cosmos, this garden, every cell in our bodies," he told the *Daily Telegraph* reporter at his estate in the English countryside. This conception fits well with the mystical philosophy underlying Sting's Yoga, a commitment easily distorted and sensationalized in his position as a world-famous practitioner. His path as both yogi and pop musician are essentially the same, "My only answer to the world's problems is the old artist's solution—love."

## Finding Peace, Gaining Release

Hard-earned after those early struggles, self-acceptance and love are among the fruits of Sting's transformation through relationship, Yoga practice, and a ruthless introspection evident in his autobiography. "I am liking myself more and more. In those early days, when I was trying to make it, I'm sure I didn't like myself," he confessed to the *Sunday Independent*. "I am happier now than I've ever been." Sting is one popular media star for whom Yoga is more than a fitness workout. Slowly over time, Yoga informed his entire life, as Sting found both personal and professional happiness. "I think you end up as your own teacher in Yoga," explained Sting to *Yoga Journal*. "I think you have to begin with a teacher, begin with a role model to guide you, but after a certain point you really are your own teacher, your own guru."

Perhaps Sting's early trials and later resolution are aptly symbolized by that surprising discovery on his Wiltshire property. In the summer of 1995 and at the behest of Trudie, workers excavated a lake and inadvertently uncovered an ancient skeleton of a ritually murdered woman. Sixteen hundred years ago, she experienced entrapment, an inner suffocation yearning for release. No doubt in camaraderie and with a wink and nod to his parents, Sting tenderly gave her a proper burial. This time, she was unbound and turned face up toward the cloudless sky with the sad but liberating sounds of bagpipes wailing in the distance. Sting stood with his love and a priest by his side. Peace at last.

CHAPTER TWENTY

20

# Water So Pure and Clear

*What is within us is also without.*
*What is without is also within.*
—Katha Upanishad

Years ago, I walked down the thoroughfare, Elisabethkai, at sunset in the beautiful alpine city of Salzberg and crossed over the bridge to the city's old section of ornate buildings facing historic squares. Peering down at the water of the River Salzach, I was surprised at how blue and clear it was in the dimmed light of dusk. The contrast with the muddier rivers back home in the Midwest was striking. Later, as I thought about how the pristine water was fed by its glaciated source in the Austrian Alps, I realized that it was an apt metaphor for how I listened to my intuitive wisdom, or *jnana*—the inner knowledge we all can access from time to time. It is a deep, elemental, instinctive, and clear knowledge that gives our lives meaning and direction.

## Energetic Wisdom

Yoga teaches us—requires us—to look within and to listen, not to the discursive mind, but to the wisdom that resides as energetic awareness in the body. Paraphrasing Patanjali in *The Yoga Sutra*, "The light of wisdom comes from perfect discipline," a discipline that begins with the body and breath only to involve more subtle aspects of mind.[1] Our bodies are great teachers, and that inner insight is a powerful tool when left uncontaminated by the turbulent waters of our mind's thoughts or those of others. If we remain attuned to that inner wisdom, it can teach and even warn us when things are not quite right in the different situations of our lives.

Listening to inner wisdom is a key to living fully. We all have had times when we have felt emotionally deadened and closed off from the world. For me, they were not happy times but were necessary for exploring my inner life directly and honestly. They were my seeds for change. The more I remain in touch with that pristine inner knowledge, the more I am open to the world and all that it can offer me. The more we are open to listening to that wisdom, the more we naturally follow the flow of our destiny, our dharma—what we are to become in this life, like a seed bursting open under just the right conditions for growth. As Patanjali reminds us, listening to our inner wisdom is also tied to synchronizing the mind and heart: "From intuition, one knows everything. From perfect discipline of the heart, one has full consciousness of one's thought."[2]

## Slaying the Inner Dragon

Such intuitive sensitivity to our inner life was the centerpiece of a well-known conversation in the mid-1980s between Joseph Campbell, renowned philosopher and historian of religion, and PBS broadcast journalist Bill Moyers. The two met for taped conversations as part of a popular television series entitled *Joseph Campbell and the Power of Myth*, which explored the universal meanings found within humankind's mythologies and their message for how to live life fully and fearlessly.

"I came to the idea of bliss," explained Campbell in his book with Moyers, "because in Sanskrit, which is the great spiritual language of the world, there are three terms that represent the brink, the jumping-off place to the ocean of transcendence: *Sat, Chit, Ananda*:"[3] Being, Consciousness, and Bliss. Of these three associations with the True Self—the primordial pure awareness of ultimate reality described in Indian Philosophy—Campbell was convinced that his own feelings of rapture or bliss were close to the original meaning in Hindu scriptures.

For Campbell, his lifelong fascination with humankind's mythological traditions was his own bliss—a personal, passionate, and intellectual quest for the universal meaning in the mythic expressions of human diversity. As Indian sages have been apt to repeat through the ages, "Truth is One but it is called by many names." The comparable stories of gods and goddesses among the world's many cultures called Campbell to a deeper awareness of himself and of the myths themselves, providing, in the "mythic hero" of great world literature, a blueprint for understanding our life's journey.

Referring to that mythic journey, Moyers asked Campbell, "How do I slay the dragon in me? What's the journey each of us has to make, what you call 'the soul's high adventure'?" Campbell replied, "Follow your bliss, find where it is, and don't be afraid to follow it." Moyers responded with another question. "Is it my work or my life?" Campbell answered, "If the work that you're doing is the work that you chose to do because you are enjoying it, that's it. But if you think, 'Oh, no! I couldn't do that!' That's the dragon locking you in. 'No, no. I couldn't be a writer,' or 'No, no. I couldn't possibly do what So-and-So is doing.'" Moyers added, "We're not going on our journey to save the world but to save ourselves."

Campbell nodded affirmatively and concluded,

> In doing that, you save the world. The influence of a vital person vitalizes, there's no doubt about it. The world without spirit is a wasteland. . . . Any world is a valid world if it's alive. The thing to do is to bring life to it, and the only way to do that is to find, in your own case, where the life is and become alive yourself. . . . Psychologically, the dragon is one's own binding of oneself to one's ego. . . . The ultimate dragon is within you, it is your ego clamping you down.[4]

## Reclaiming Joie de Vivre

Joseph Campbell's notion of "following your bliss" became a cliché well before the yoga explosion ignited throughout the country, especially among the segment of Americans attuned to spiritual things and to examining their inner lives and opportunities for personal transformation. Campbell was not referring to the indescribably delicious bliss known to some yogis, which is an actual psycho-physiological experience, nor perhaps to its original meaning. Rather, his words referred to how we must listen to our inner wisdom unencumbered by ego or that which we or others *think* is right or best for us, including the opinions of parents, teachers, friends, intimates, or co-workers. We must listen beyond the dictates of our seemingly solid identities to that which is fundamentally and intimately true about ourselves, to our *svabhava*, or inner being—that which scholar Ravi Ravindra calls "the lord seated in the heart."[5]

Sometimes others' common-sense advice is right on the mark. But often our challenges in following *our* path—the one with heart—have to do with first acknowledging what makes *us* feel most fully alive. Only then can we recognize the difference between confused perceptions, expectations, judgments, or attachments on the one hand and what we know feels right on the other. Lastly, we must find the courage to act—to follow our bliss, or life's purpose, to its natural, evolving endpoint. Depending on our situations, this may demand a dramatic change in a job, relationship, or where we call home. At other times, the courage to change requires fine tweaking. It ultimately depends on how off course we have been from where our true bliss lies.

Poets, artists, contemplatives, and members of other thoughtful professions create lives where finding their bliss is the field for their creativity. "Most people are concerned with other things," explained Campbell. "But most people living in that realm of what might be called 'occasional concerns' have the capacity that is waiting to be awakened to move to this other field. I know, I have seen it happen."[6] Perhaps the *Brihadaranyaka Upanishad* captures this truth most succinctly: "You are what your deep, driving desire is. As your desire is, so is your will. As your will is, so is your deed. As your deed is, so is your destiny."

So how do we recognize our bliss—our desire, dharma, or duty to live our destinies? We know it by how it manifests in our lives. There is nothing else we would rather be doing and nothing that fuels such passion for living while taking us deeper into understanding our life's mysteries; it may be Yoga, art, writing, nature, music, travel, or teaching—whatever touches and informs us most deeply and viscerally. Unlike an unhealthy attachment, our bliss is known by the sweet fruit that it bears: love, joy, openness, well-being, and a positive regard for the world. In other words, that fruit is joie de vivre.

While all these avenues can cultivate our inner wisdom that provides the seeds for our transformation, they differ in the breadth and depth to which they do so. Application of Patanjali's pragmatic and meditative roadmap, the eight limbs of Yoga, ensures that our awareness can unfold naturally through the practices of ethical restraint and observance, asana and breath work, and stages of sensory withdrawal, concentration, meditation, and absorption. The eight limbs provide the well-worn energetic pathway by which we can find our bliss and feel fully alive in the body. Those of Tantric persuasion might add other practices like mantra recitation, deity worship, and pilgrimages to sacred places. Regardless of the Yogic path we take, we can learn to live in the present moment, clearly seeing what lies closest to our hearts.

## Invisible Waters Flow

After dinner on that starry September night back in Salzberg, I walked through the streets of its old town and past the tourist shops that called out to my pocketbook. In crossing back over the river, I now knew that the darkened waters were naturally pure and clear. Yet that awareness was based on my experience—my memory of the river to which I could always return as long as I remained open and sensitive to it. Similarly, we can continue to cultivate our intuitive wisdom—becoming aware of that which was unconscious—and can be reminded that it is within us at the very point that we seem blind or unable to recognize it. Over the years, Yoga has become my continuous cultivation of that inner source which is fuel for finding my bliss. It actually *is* that bliss, where our life's journey and destination are really the very same thing. And for the millions of new yoga practitioners, Yoga offers the opportunity to become theirs, not as a unique activity but as a chain of lifelong transformations.

CHAPTER TWENTY-ONE

# Elephant-Headed

The power of ancient story is no myth. We benefit from understanding the great mythologies of premodern civilizations and mining them for their deeper meaning. Their wise and symbolic teachings guide us toward a greater appreciation of our personal challenges and opportunities and offer us beacons of wisdom that can light up and enliven our purpose of fostering growth and rebirth. Myth is yet another resource for svadhyaya—serious self-study and observation—in a Yogic legacy that calls for us to examine ourselves more deeply.

Contrary to contemporary secular thought, our lives need not be viewed as random accidents lacking meaningful and essentially spiritual lessons. Our lives have intrinsic meaning informed by our life purpose, our dharma. Carl Jung, Joseph Campbell, and others believe that mythology holds underlying messages about the human psyche and the purpose of human life. Jean Shinoda Bolen, M.D., conveyed this idea beautifully in her bestselling classic *Goddesses in Everywoman*. Through her writings and clinical practice, she explored how gods and goddesses symbolize common themes or archetypes that men and women embody at different phases in their lives. Virgin goddesses, like Athena, are independent and self-directed to cultivate what is most meaningful to them. Hera and other more vulnerable deities seek attachment or engagement and grow through their suffering and victimization. Alchemical goddesses, like Aphrodite, are intense, sensual, and always open to their transformations. Yet each archetype embodies their seeds of metamorphosis.

The Indian gods and goddesses that permeate Yoga's wisdom teachings do the same. As particular energies, their mythic stories beckon practitioners to explore their deeper meanings, unfolding to inform a path of personal progress. Often involving grotesque images of divinities, Hindu myths explain conventional matters like birth, death, and rebirth which symbolize our life journeys as mythic heroes seeking a sense of freedom, release from suffering, or our own alchemical transmutations.

In Hinduism, masculine and feminine energies unfold as stories of how to confront challenges, including the artful handling of beginnings and endings. Finding a new career, home, or intimate relationship—some of our most profound and surprising events—call for courage and insight and allow us to learn from the myths of the great world civilizations. While chanting mantras in Sanskrit acts to purify mind and heart, full application of a mythic story to our lives is similarly instructive, since it points us in the direction of the source of all sacred language of the East—acting in concert with our higher self. Practitioners of Yoga can tap these intelligent energies to aid their own transformations or those of others, as portals to higher realization.

## Applying Myth to Life

Each of us has our own serpentine journey of ill-health or healing. Years ago, I had separated from my wife and moved to a nearby city to gain perspective as well as emotional and physical distance from a difficult marital situation. I was also trying to complete my doctoral training. Feeling personally demoralized and depressed, financially strapped and intellectually challenged, I was also restricted geographically: Finding a job outside the state would have meant losing joint custody and regular contact with my young daughter. I was trapped and unable to generate momentum to break free of my emotional claustrophobia. Looking back now, I realize that the myth of Ganesha is a blueprint for how I emerged, and how others can emerge, from personal malaise.[1]

At that time in my life, I had retreated into an impotent phase of physical weakness and emotional numbness. For years, I became ill with intermittent, month-long fevers that allopathic physicians could not precisely diagnose using their testing procedures and disease categories. I was weak, lacking that zest for life that characterizes the happy, energetic person. My body felt heavy, or *tamsic*, in Yogic terms, and I was stuck physically and emotionally, a personal and yet all-too-universal form of dukkha. Knowing that I had to break free—an essential meaning of renunciation in Yoga—led me to understand more fully how I could embody a sacred story as mythic hero of my life.

I had run across the various myths of the Indian god, Ganesha, many years earlier, in doing research on Hinduism. Elephant gods are popular figures throughout Asia and are said to derive from Indian Tantra, illustrating how creative, wrathful, and protective energies manifest as potentiality for transformation and rebirth. Royina Grewal has pointed out, in *The Book of Ganesha*, that Tibetan Tantric texts even identify him with *bodhisattvas*, or enlightened beings of compassion, of whom the Dalai Lama is a living incarnation.[2] Ganesha, also known as Ganapati, is revered throughout India as the "remover of obstacles" and is symbolically important at any phase of our lives, but especially when we undertake a new adventure or want to learn from the loss of anything we cherish.

Myths about Ganesha attribute his physical condition as half elephant, half human, to different origins. The actions of Shiva—the supreme ascetic, phallic god of transformation and lord of Yoga—are used in some myths to explain his son Ganesha's status as a major god of the Hindu pantheon as well as his unique physical condition. Goddess Parvati—Shiva's wife and Ganesha's mother—and the elephant-headed one are often depicted as seated beside Shiva. On one level, all that we need to overcome a critical life situation seems embodied in their images: Shiva as potency for change, or kama, that primal seed of desire reflected in creative action; Parvati as nurturing, protective, and magnetizing energy; and the unplanned outcome of their interaction—the wise guardianship as symbolized by Ganesha.

His creation story varies widely across the Indian subcontinent, with explanations of his fate coming from the *Shiva-Purana,* ancient Vedic scriptures. As one popular story has it, the goddess Parvati created him from the perfumed paste on her body, breathing life into the boy and instructing him to act as guard, with mace in hand, as she and her companions bathed. Stirred from his meditation, Shiva amorously sought his wife but was halted by Ganesha. Enraged, Shiva beheaded him. The shocked Parvati became so disconsolate that the couple had a momentous fight. In resolution, Shiva ordered his celestial attendants to travel northward to bring him the head of the first sleeping animal they encountered. The head of an elephant was severed, transported, and transplanted by Shiva onto Ganesha's body. He named the transformed boy Ganapati, commander of his celestial forces, or *ganas*.

Ganesha's mythic story of creation, death, and rebirth finds Shiva's pure desire yearning for fulfillment but leading to aggression and conflict. How commonly do our own frustrations at being stuck—at not reaching an important goal to which we strive—lead to destructive expression? How often do our desires lead to clinging and suffering? Is closing down physically and emotionally just another form of aggression, only pointed inward? How can our compassionate, creative energies be redirected to find meaningful resolutions to such difficulties? Real transformation demands that we, like Shiva, cut decisively through that which stands in our way. When a critical life event cuts us down, the opportunity for our transformation naturally arises. The sheer excitement of that field of open possibilities fuels tremendous creativity to reshape our lives. Ignoring, squandering, or misusing this opportunity can feel like such great loss.

## BECOMING GANESHA

Other transformational symbolism is inherent in statuary found throughout India of the bulbous-bellied elephant god riding on a rodent, with powerful weaponry held firmly in his many hands. The elephant is by nature strong, gentle, loyal, intelligent, and affectionate—qualities we need to turn our lives artfully in new directions. We need strength and determination, tapas, to take action when the time is auspicious, when the iron is hot; a kind and fair resolve toward ourselves and others if we make mistakes; a loyalty to what we stand for, to what we need to be happy, and to the process of getting "there" from "here"; and commitment to ahimsa, as manifested in a gentle and tender heart, in light of what the unknown has to offer.

Yet something even more essential is required to turn our lives in new directions. Both myth and statuary ask us to fully accept the elephant god and to find the wisdom or truth that lies beyond the surface, behind external appearances, and beyond our physical bodies. Ganapati's most noticeable trait is his head, that great symbol of strength and intellectual prowess. Honoring him implies that we attempt to tame our runaway intellects and monkey minds through inner discrimination, seeing situations clearly and considering our options wisely. With those great ears, we learn to flap away obstacles to our happiness.

A year after my divorce, I recognized that meaningful opportunities for change would only manifest if I underwent serious self-study, or svadhyaya. Otherwise, I would continue the same old habitual patterns that never brought real happiness. Self-study meant, for me, exploring meditation and yoga. And I did, with a zeal for regular practice. At weekend meditation retreats, I learned to quiet my mind; to watch thoughts rise and fall without chasing them; and to rest in that gap between thoughts so situations arose naturally and my inner wisdom informed action with a more tender, honest, and open heart.

My blossoming daily yoga practice at home was motivated initially by a wish to overcome my "energy illness" and to push it away. My perspective evolved with time and a growing commitment to meditation. Eventually, during a personal audience with Buddhist nun Pema Chödrön, I realized that I had come slowly to accept—even to embrace—the recurrent onset of my illness. My health and healing yoga, now coupled with meditation, slid toward Yoga as I concentrated more on centering awareness on my breath and synchronizing my mind and body through movement. As I walked my newfound path of self-discovery, sometimes in utter exhaustion, I eventually reclaimed my energy. The fevers abated with time, never to appear again.

## Embodied Myth

From the Indian standpoint, for Hinduism and Buddhism alike, stilling the reflective mind is key to cultivating awareness in any situation. The many-armed Ganesha often rides on a rodent—seen scurrying about like our wandering, restless minds—which he symbolically subjugates underfoot, showing us clearly how to handle situations wisely and artfully. And I was now facing new life situations. Would a new romantic relationship be grounded in something substantial or be driven primarily by physical attraction or lust? Would opening a new business help me "follow my bliss," or would it be my desperate attempt to escape a bad work situation?

Now I could see the field of choices before me and a slow-growing sense of abundance and opportunity, symbolized by Ganesha's bulbous belly. Perhaps that belly is the most esoteric of all his traits. Draped with a snake—symbolic of primordial Shakti energy tied to our freedom and happiness—Ganesha artfully digests all experiences without exception or judgment, according to Grewal. Ganesha is nourished by the entire process of our lifelong transformations, which can include the rising of kundalini from muladhara chakra at the base of the spine.

Ganesha, then, is instructive of how to handle impending situations—learning to hold our regal seats like Indian rajas on the backs of pachyderms and not to react to situations reflexively, whether with heightened excitement, strong emotional energy, or sexual desire. I had slowly learned to sit up and observe, to find my still point, and to feel the rough texture of any emotional pull without racing to reach an outcome that created more trouble for me. I had learned to create space—that perceptual gap between initial impulse and an imagined resolution. Yet my desire to transform myself was the source of my rebirth. Within five years, and with more than a little auspicious luck, I completed my doctoral dissertation, found my life partner, and took a job offering stability that ensured daily contact with my daughter.

Ganesha's hands are a cogent reminder of that time for me now. His hand gestures or mudras denote the granting of wishes and the dispelling of fear. Both hopes and fears are associated with our attachment, the clinging to an anticipated future or comfortable past, leading us to flee or fight and not to hold our ground in the present moment. Working with our hopes and fears through cultivation of one-pointed concentration (*ekagrata*) in sitting meditation and through that "meditation in motion" called Yoga results in greater openness and acceptance of self and our life situation. My Yoga practice allowed me to move beyond perceptions of situations as thorny obstacles that could have bound me to a preconceived notion of a desired or feared result.

"Moving beyond" revealed that my perception of obstacles—including my illness—was closely tied to the grasping quality of my ego. As we release our clinging to a preconceived or desired outcome, we naturally dissolve any sense of obstacle to happiness. That prickly thorn called the lower mind, or controlling ego, gives way to the healing salve that is our higher self—our natural, spontaneous state of wisdom.

The weaponry in Ganesha's many hands includes objects necessary for such a metamorphosis. His pointed, prodding rod produces movement, generating our first steps onto the adventurous roads we are to travel. Tapas is our enthusiastic determination to move toward an unknown destination of greater intimacy, commitment and self-revelation. While Ganesha's short-handled ax cuts our bondage to desire, his noose draws it closer with its bound knot. Rather than avoiding those things that disrupt the stability of our minds, we are asked to find that point of inner awareness from which to observe and feel desire, allowing us to discriminate between what will be suitable and healthy for us and others, and what will not. And while at times I may fail, I have learned that it is my commitment to and reaffirmation of this principle that counts the most.

## Mythic Recipe

Ganesha's myth and symbolism provide a recipe for freeing ourselves to succeed at any mythic adventure and provide all the ingredients to triumph over adversity. We may have different strengths and find varied solutions to our particular life challenges. But the ingredients remain the same: quieting the mind to see the situation clearly; finding courage to generate movement from inertia; acknowledging desire's embrace; doing what we intuitively know is right in situations pregnant with possibility; and cultivating openness, fearlessness, and joy by giving up attachment to outcome. Surrendering to Ganesha is an especially useful teaching, since every moment of our lives is a transformative opportunity—a new beginning, arrival, or birth as well as an ending, departure, or death. When we apply this myth's deeper meanings, we honor that elephant-headed god on the altar of our lives. We become one with Ganapati, open to whatever life and death will offer us.

CHAPTER TWENTY-TWO

# Last Breath

*A moment of love may seem like a small thing,*
*but at the moment of death that love will be everything.*
—Babaji's Kriya Yoga Ashram

She gasped for air—the ocean sound of ujayi with the mouth open. But there was no energy with an out-breath, only the sobs of my sisters in the background. This moment, this precious moment, was our last breath together.

As I stared at her, breath no longer animated her body. The woman before me was my life's constancy; we were together in both birth and death. Once a buoyant and happy, loving but stern taskmaster, she had morphed before my eyes into a stiffened slab of white shriveled flesh. But this moment of her passing had a peculiar sense of achievement, for it was the gasp of goodbye and the kiss of moving on. Then, I recalled what Ram Dass had written in *Still Here*: "Death is our greatest challenge as well as our greatest spiritual opportunity."[1] Moments later, I got up from the foot of her bed and walked down the nursing home corridor to cry. Collecting myself, I called my daughter to tell her the news. After four days in the hospital, I told her, my mom had passed.

I loved my mother as most sons do. I did not quite understand her world, as she could not quite fathom mine. She was the aproned, traditional Czech with a grammar-school education. I was the T-shirted, jaded university-trained professional. Her world and mine were more than generations apart—Lawrence Welk meets the Dalai Lama, Suburbia meets Soho, or Limbo meets Lennon. My Catholic upbringing, which was so important to her, had sown seeds of my critical thinking that eventually turned the church on its head. The mop-top sixties and hang-loose seventies birthed a conscientious objector, social scientist, meditator, and yoga teacher. During all these changes, my mother remained the faith-driven arbiter of right and wrong and of simple views of how life ought to be lived, like the commandments etched in marble in a parish sacristy.

Despite our differences, we met somewhere in the middle over the decades. Our weekly talks revolved around relationships and old times held in common and were always couched by bookends made of those simple words, "I love you." We understood those words like two good friends on a park bench who cannot speak the same language yet recognize the simple affectionate gaze in each other's eyes or like two fish flip-flopping separately on the shore to find the water that sustains them both. But her last breath called out to me now, like the sound of love momentarily interrupted. Breath, the outward manifestation of the life force, bound my mother and me together as it binds us all.

The infinitely creative energy that rides on our breaths was the common denominator of our differences. My mother was born in bed in a rural Wisconsin hamlet where only Bohemian was spoken. That was her world for the first sixteen years, as faith, food, and family served as an impregnable string connecting her birth and death like pearls of different moments in time. So much had passed between us, so many beginnings and endings—the tenderness of a mother holding her only son as he fumbles with her fingers; communion, confirmation, and moral criticism; fits of adolescent irrationality testing invisible boundaries; confusing years of war, contention, peace, and love; the prodigal return with a grandchild with whom she spends hours crawling on the floor; her tears of disappointment at my divorce; and then twenty years of synchrony.

Ram Dass explains that "the moment of death does not necessarily transform us; we die, after all, as who we are, no better or worse, no wiser or more ignorant. We each bring to the moment of our passing the summation of all that we've lived and done."[2] That also applies to those who are at our passage into the Great Unknown, for they share in our summation as part of the living.

Our eyes did not meet at my mother's passing. She fell into a coma four days earlier. On that first day, I held her wrinkled hand and asked if she recognized my voice. I felt the squeeze of sweet affirmation where words again failed. I whispered in her ear and into her heart, "Say your prayers." Prayers to Jesus and Mary and Joseph were never far from her lips. That would be our last audible communication. The days passed in vigil at my mother's bedside until that warm September Sunday morning. A priest and nun came and went, when she would have nodded off and struggled to stay awake at Mass. My sisters and I awaited her death.

I sat with eyes closed in meditation, visualizing Jesus above her bed with intense rays of white light and love pouring down onto her. I slowly breathed in and out from my heart to hers and back again very slowly. There was that last gasp for air. I opened my eyes to see this frail, sweet old woman with mouth widened and stilled. I closed my eyes again and returned to my breath. Then, I felt the tingling of her energy, of her wind, of prana on my body. It hovered for a few seconds, and it was gone. This woman who had given me life gave me a last, lasting memory like none other. At his own mother's death, Ram Dass felt she was like a person in a collapsing building. "Our connection seems to be independent of the building," he told her. "You'll go on even though your body won't. And we'll stay connected."[3] I know what he meant.

Thoughts of my mother now drift through my mind like so much decaying wood on the beach, bobbing up and down with the rolling tide as she swims over that vast ocean of love. They are memories accompanied by a tender joy and sad realization of how fleeting they all are. This is death's bittersweet quality, always in the background, to remind me of my own impermanence as I wait patiently at the distant shore to join her in my own time, with the affectionate eyes of an old friend.

* * *

Meditation on death and at death, with focused attention to prana, is among Tantra's great gifts to humankind.[4] Yet it feels more important to me to be fully present for a dying person at the moment of their passing—to hold them in our hearts—than it is to feel their energy as they leave this earth. We have met death, our old friend, many times before, according to the Yogic worldview. While our deaths are said to be precious opportunities to gain awareness of our true nature—the luminous, blissful, and clear light of our True Self—they are also openings for both the dying and the living. For yogis, life is the cause of our deaths, and death the cause of our lives.

Whenever I live my Yoga, I am also "dying my Yoga." The very same principles and practices that guide me in finding peace and happiness in this life are the ones that will aid my own exiting or that of someone I love—honoring my commitments; having a regular, fully engaged practice; working with my mind and sensory world through meditation; opening my heart through mantra and visualization; and engaging with the energy on a slow and deepened breath. These are my priorities in living my Yoga, regardless of who or what I have become, personally or professionally. When I work with my body, mind, and heart through Yoga practice, I more easily open to others, no matter how distant their lives seem from my own. Aiding them even in the simplest way as they face unusual or difficult situations is a lasting gift, born of love.

Our relationship to Yoga—entered with curiosity and wonder, fed by compassion and determination, and nurtured by an energetic joie de vivre—involves a gentle warriorship of unconditional love that can be taken out into the world, whether at a birth or at the side of a dying loved one. When we commit to living Yoga, we are willing to take on the constant challenge of moving at our edges, at our borders. We are challenged to enter discomforting situations that test our willingness to free ourselves by giving up attachment to identities that are transitory and will perish with our bodies and by giving up the clinging to situations that only bring unhappiness. In so doing, we experience Yoga's great promise to us. It has much less to do with mastering gymnastic poses and much more to do with learning to work directly with life's energetic quality—the common denominator of our differences—through breath, that liberating and healing force which is our natural connection with the world.

CONCLUSION

# The Frog under Our Mat

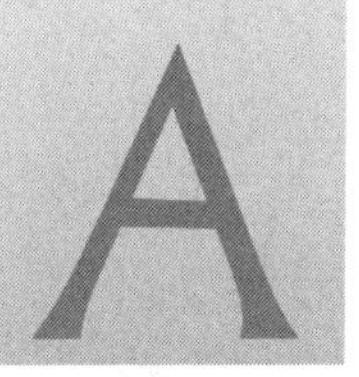

After completing the first draft of this book, I had a curious dream in which a frog situated himself on the brick patio at my back door. He neither surprised nor frightened me as I observed him with equanimity. He was merely poised at the door, ready to gain entry into an orderly, domesticated world from the untamed gardens of my backyard in spring. Upon waking, I thought of how fitting this image was—how I am transformed through Yoga as a path; how a wild, undisciplined, and often unyielding body, mind, and heart are tamed, redirected, and opened to invite entry; and how this process of closing and opening, contracting and releasing, seems endless.

Our dreams are often sources of creativity and insight. For some, they are considered forms of communication between different parts of ourselves, pregnant with meaning from the unconscious. Unlocking that meaning increases self-awareness, whether their symbolism is viewed as inherent to the dream itself or is projected onto the dream by a now-awake dreamer. In Eastern traditions, there are practices associated with Sleep Yoga which involve meditative exploration through lucid dreaming. We, as "dreamers," learn to influence our dreams, piercing the subtle layers separating the conscious and unconscious.

While there was no conscious influence, I was certain there was a deeper meaning to my dream image. The frog's intrinsic qualities are symbols of self-exploration and transformation in so many cultural, religious, and intellectual traditions. This ancient amphibian inhabits all kinds of terrain from deserts to tropics and is adaptable to both land and water. Perhaps we are most familiar with the image of the frog submerged in his pond, except for those bulbous eyes and nose exposed in the moonlight.

The frog is closely associated with these water and lunar elements, common metaphors for the unconscious in dream therapy. To survive, he keeps his body moist—in contact with the water that sustains him—and changes colors while remaining camouflaged. Frogs are tied to svadhisthana and the genital region in the Yogic geography of the body—the energy center of the water element manifesting as potency, creativity, connection, and desire. And frogs do exert great energy to mate, croaking their songs of love or, as expressed in the Vedas, of praise for the coming of the life-sustaining spring rains.

Many masters over the millennia have suggested that most central to the Yogic path is personal metamorphosis—like the movement of egg to tadpole to frog, from frog to dragon-slaying prince—in bringing to the surface hidden truth that transforms the practitioner. Long ago, Swami Sivananda noted, in an encyclopedic list of dream symbols, that the harmless nature of the frog portends a favorable or successful outcome.[1] Swami Vishnu Tirtha used the imagery of a frog to explain physical manifestations of that rarified kundalini energy rising in the body.[2] Scholar of myth Joseph Campbell stressed the frog's symbolism in more Jungian terms, as that which is unconscious rising to awareness, thereby transforming the dreamer into something truly pure and beautiful.[3] Fully accepting ourselves where we are at this very moment, warts and all, is the necessary first step in our personal metamorphoses through Yoga.

In Yogic traditions, it is said that when the student is ready, the teacher appears. Central to the transformative process of our lives is matching our inner readiness, determination, and intuition to walk down the Yogic path with a guide who can point out the way through the thicket. Without both of these necessary elements, we are likely to thrash in our personal lily ponds of confusion, misdirection, hope, and fear. Employing tapas without svadhiyaya—the love and discipline for walking the path without studying the image exposed in the mirror-like wisdom of a gifted teacher—manifests as an unnecessary dead end of wasted time and energy.

This book has described how love fuels our determination to practice Yoga, deepens our relationship to it, and manifests what is possible through it—namely, a healing wisdom energy. Its stories, each in their own way, embody that theme. They remind us that external appearances are deceptive in the same way that Indian philosophy informs us of *maya*, the seemingly illusory world we inhabit. All we must do is scratch the surface to find that things are not as they appear: the unassuming yoga teacher ends up a spiritually gifted being; an international pop star is anything but a superficial practitioner; the confused student transforms himself by living out an ancient mythic message; a travel getaway spawns healing more than rest and relaxation; a class for the obese fosters love and acceptance, not weight loss; an unlikely friendship brings out-of-the-ordinary insight; and death's door opens, rather than shuts, on intimacy. These stories tap our innate wisdom to see what is invisible in the visible and what is essential in the ordinary. I hope I have lit a transformative spark in the reader in the same way that Yoga lived as a holistic path lends its power to all those who walk it.

## THE CHALLENGE FOR AMERICAN YOGA

This book has also been about a fast-moving transformation that can either feed or starve personal metamorphosis. Yoga's future in

America relies upon the intentions and motivations of those who practice and who apply its deeper teachings to their experiences and to the lives of those they touch. Paradoxically, it may be yoga's popularity with the mainstream—for fitness or health—that leads many more people to rediscover its spiritual center. It is just as likely, though, that those attracted to yoga for more physical reasons may not look more deeply, altering and narrowing how the public views the practice in the long run.

With its new or refashioned forms, we cannot avoid the truth that Yoga is being repackaged. Such change would be healthy if only Yoga's wisdom center remained intact and its deeper practices were clearly visible, accessible, and transmitted to committed students. Yoga's public persona, as in more extreme forms of fitness yoga, feels disassociated at times from its philosophical origins. While most yoginis may not want anything more than to feel fit or balanced, those seeking growth also need their avenue easily available and intentions respected, regardless of current market demand.

If teachers grounded in the deeper message of Yoga are not available or do not share what they know, Srivatsa Ramaswami predicts "the subject will die because every following generation will know less and less. And the lack of knowledge could be filled with innovations of novices, leading to corruption or the art dying itself."[4]

Yoga's spread to the mainstream amounts to its secularization, as the essence that was once its bedrock is undercut by media culture, commercialism, and medicalization stressing the physical effects of asana practice. These developments, adherents claim, are positive by bringing health and healing to millions of more people. Yet it is problematic when they are not fueled by the deeper understanding of what creates human suffering, by the wisdom central to Yoga's message for humankind, or by its essentially transcendental focus.

In some sense, maintaining its wisdom center may have always been the challenge for Yoga in America, with its frog-like adaptability.

Maybe it is only that this trend has accelerated and is now more clearly seen or more pervasive. In a society which prides itself on openness and tolerance, a despiritualized fitness yoga—one less clearly rooted and having fewer spiritually gifted teachers as guides—more easily gains popularity with the mainstream. While fighting flab, managing stress, or strengthening an injured limb meet important personal needs, they do little to instruct us on how to live and how to "live Yoga" as a form of cultural rebellion.

If this transformative spirituality is not protected from the broad secularizing influences discussed in this book, there is nothing to slow the movement toward an equally superficial understanding of the Yogic meaning system and of the way it explains the world and the human search for happiness. Once any meaning system loses its original message, visibility, or influence on a societal level, there is less sharing or learning firsthand from its teachings. As a consequence, we students are simultaneously burdened *and* unmoored, left to believe what we want, independent of any external guidance or deeper understanding. We are adrift to be influenced by the superficial, commercial winds that blow from Hollywood through the plasma screens.

Yoga, to be authentic, does not need to be practiced with sitar music in the background, wearing loincloths, or taught by someone of Indian descent chanting "Om." These are the cultural window dressings of a stereotyped spiritual yoga. After all, truth is truth regardless of culture, race, or sect. However, if some civilizations have held closely to the wellspring of wisdom and compassion through inner technologies tested over the millennia, *they* need a continuous forum. And *we* need them to continue to inform *us* about how to see clearly, surrounded as we are by all the confusion, aggression, and desires of a world out of balance.

An illustrative parallel for Yoga's future may well be the issue of global warming. It is invisible to us day-to-day except for singular, catastrophic and well-publicized events. Yet its gradual, long-term impact upon humanity will be horrific. Global warming will never be seriously addressed if scientists, citizenry, politicians, and industrialists deny its existence or fail to band together to counter those committed foremost to advancing the interests of commerce and the mindless consumption which are themselves the source of the crisis. Certainly, economic sacrifice will be necessary for our collective well-being.

So it is with Yoga, a five-thousand-year-old "ice shield" that embodies a promise of transformation. Perhaps those who love Yoga are obliged to make their voices heard whenever it undergoes this type of fundamental change, to make not just their personal but our social transformation possible. This obligation demands openness to experience as well as hopefulness about Yoga's future. Otherwise, it will not be worth the time to faithfully pass on its truths to future generations. Without Yoga's essence preserved—its "arctic glacial shelf"—it is melted down under the heated pressure of commercial interests. One solution is to more consciously dedicate ourselves—personally and collectively—to preserving Yoga's long-term well-being, just as Indian practitioners did in the nineteenth century as part of their country's independence movement.

## Acting for Self-Transformation

Our own mythic quests through Yoga do not require journeys to India, although visiting its many holy sites and practice centers may provide us with energy, power, and insight. Rather, we might simply look for teachers who live Yoga and who match our need to address the mind, body, and heart in class. Outside of class, Yoga can enliven us in the simplest of ways—living in moderation, practicing asanas regularly, and reflecting on the yamas and niyamas. Yoga means being mindful of our breaths, of how we sit at desks, of what sensations arise in our bodies without judgment. Living Yoga also means taking up mind training—meditation practice—and studying its psychology and philosophy.

In our own parts of the country and in our communities, we can also seek pockets of practitioners for whom Yoga remains a wellspring for a richer and deeper practice beyond gymnastic competency. Checking with yoga teachers we know or leafing through local holistic publications is a good first step in locating these practitioners. We may find that they practice with gentleness and good cheer, chant the names of theistic divinities, or celebrate with love and joy the formless Energy-Consciousness that permeates everything. We need not convert to an exotic or foreign-born religion but only take the opportunity to participate in a more inclusive spirituality. All we need is to discover, experience, and acknowledge what feels best for us and to consider practicing with regularity.

The retreat centers and ashrams around the country act as friendly seedbeds from which a more robust Yoga can revitalize, helping us to create or maintain our practice. There, we are more likely to find America's living masters of Yoga from whom we can take intensives, programs, and workshops that hone our skillfulness while establishing supportive relationships that may last a lifetime. If we live too far from these restorative resources or if our own finances are limited, the Internet provides access to many excellent books, magazines, tapes, and CDs that can deepen our understanding and our practice (*Yoga Journal*'s site offers a wide range of materials). The Web also furnishes a dispersed community of dedicated individuals interested in sharing their own stories of transformation, which can keep us motivated to practice.

In the final analysis, these are not prescriptive measures, only ideas for deepening our practices and strengthening Yoga in America.

## Acting for Social Transformation

And what can be done on a societal level? Any rebalancing act in America will demand more focused attention to this issue from the spiritually engaged segment of today's "Yoga industry leaders"—the many gifted teachers, their informed practitioners, national organizations, writers, publishers, entrepreneurs, and studio owners dedicated to preserving its wise teachings. To widen the dialogue, national conferences might choose the contemporary yoga scene as one of their discussion topics for those dedicated to transformative consciousness. Supporting preservation projects—like the Yoga Research and Education Center's translations and publications, in conjunction with Babaji's Kriya Yoga Ashram—will ensure future access to ancient Yogic texts in jeopardy of being lost or destroyed.

Perhaps rebalancing calls for the Yoga Alliance, tireless advocate for teachers and training programs, to set more extensive requirements for organizations in its broadening registry, so that teachers become more firmly grounded in the philosophical bases and practices of the path. In the context of the eight limbs, this would include a strong background in meditation practice. If teachers do not have such experience, how can we expect students to understand its importance? While respecting diversity, the Alliance can also help formalize the distinction between Yoga as ancient holistic discipline and yoga as physically based workout, to provide national clarity for practitioners and the public at large.

Following the lead of educational accreditation bodies, class offerings at centers around the country could simply be reviewed to create a national guide to places offering practices that go beyond asanas. Those centers based on spiritual principles might consider loosely affiliating themselves to explore the mutual benefits of collaboration. The Kripalu Center for Yoga and Health and the Shambhala Mountain Center began such a dialogue in 2001, and their experience could be used as both springboard and sounding board for future possibilities. Rebalancing Yoga might be further nurtured by establishing a national center which intends to preserve its history and traditions in America by tracking trends of what is currently a highly decentralized and consumer-driven growth industry.

An especially important development of the past few decades has been how the spiritual commitment of Yoga practitioners has informed their professional training. These professionals are Yoga's important middle ground between tradition and postmodernity. Acting as exemplars of Yoga's power to transform, they bring the path into everyday life and provide it as a resource for others. Some are themselves students of those experts, or "dispellers of darkness," known as gurus. These professionals include the presidents, scholars-in-residence, and medical directors at retreat centers; program coordinators and senior students at ashrams; and psychologists, physicians, teachers, counselors, social workers, yoga therapists, and other helping professionals working around the country.

These are today's "Yogic Vanguard," maintaining its integrity as a transformative path—its hidden soul under the mat—while assimilating it into cultural life as something more than mere fitness workout stripped of deeper practices. This Vanguard also includes chant masters who refrain from becoming performers; rock stars who live Yoga and share their commitment with their fans; and therapists who are informed rather than governed by the mainstream medical worldview. The Vanguard is magazine editors and book authors who talk frankly about that which protects their sales; and studio owners walking their spiritual talk and, where necessary, sacrificing part of their livelihoods to do it. The Vanguard includes newly trained teachers who integrate spirituality into their classes and extend it to groups who do not know of its hidden potential; students who engage with ethical precepts and selfless service in daily life while having fun practicing; and all who remain mindful while focusing attention on their breaths.

The Vanguard is comprised of all those practitioners for whom Yoga's magic heals, purifies, and makes whole again, and who tell of its power. They are the single most important resource for ideas and actions that will revitalize Yoga in America. Since social change demands collective action, their networking at national meetings may help to generate a rebirth.

## A Heartfelt Aspiration

My hope for Yoga practice is simple: May its timeless teachings be preserved, honored, and strengthened, and may this become our shared dream and intentional restoration—our *mandukasana*, or frog pose—practiced together. In the process, the purity of our motivations as practitioners is essential. If we practice Yoga to live in the present moment by synchronizing mind and movement as a meditation in action, wisdom will naturally arise. If we practice Yoga to cultivate an open heart so that we can be filled with a love artfully transmitted to others, this too will manifest. If we do both of these things while dedicating the merits of our practices to all those we touch while gently challenging them to "live and die Yoga," then our efforts will eventually tap Yoga's potential to transform the world.

May we pass our positive intention along, forged by the fire of personal experience and guided by those who have come before us with greater wisdom and compassion than our own. May all of us—regardless of why, how, and where we practice in America's yoga subculture—be happy, healthy, at our ease, safe, and free from suffering. May we embody these qualities before, during, and after asana practice. May we remain gentle, open, vulnerable, and sensitive to all that this world offers. If we can do *these* things, the superficial will become truly meaningful, and Yoga will continue to be what it has always been—a path for unifying mind and body and heart that offers a simple, peaceful, and profound way to change lives for the better.

Social recovery and personal metamorphosis begin by examining our own perceptions and intentions and our own expectations and judgments of ourselves. It cannot be otherwise. Only in this way do we begin to gain freedom from clinging to past deficiency where we are never good enough, strong enough, straight enough, long enough, wise enough, or young enough just to be who and how and what we are at this very moment. The natural outcome of our transformation is happiness, at peace with ourselves and the world. This is Yoga's promise, what Krishnamacharya once called India's greatest gift. We must not waste it on what it was never meant to be.

Om Shanti. Peace.

APPENDIX A

# What Kind of Practitioner Are You?

This is meant to be a fun exercise to make simple distinctions among types of practitioners. Circle an answer for each of these true/false statements, and score yourself below.

1. I do yoga because it makes me feel good. T F
2. I love doing yoga to a contemporary rock or jazz beat. T F
3. Feeling more alive and self-aware motivates me to go deeper in yoga. T F
4. I practice to gain physical relief or to heal myself physically. T F
5. I prefer a fitness center or workout environment to a yoga studio or center. T F
6. I have a regular meditation practice that complements my asana practice. T F
7. I read up on specific health benefits of the poses I do. T F
8. Looking good in class is important to me. T F
9. *Yoga Journal* is my bible; I am an avid reader. T F
10. The sacredness of living things motivated me to become a vegetarian. T F

11. A health professional's recommendations partly influence me to practice. T F
12. I often read yoga books by spiritual teachers, masters, or scholars. T F
13. My body's appearance and muscle tone motivate me to practice. T F
14. Body therapies in addition to yoga help me address a physical issue. T F
15. I practice yoga with workout goals in mind. T F
16. I consciously apply the yamas and niyamas to my life. T F
17. I am very motivated to improve my postures. T F
18. I cannot tell swastikasana from sirsasana. T F
19. I practice because yoga definitely prevents illness and injury. T F
20. I never discuss doing my yoga with family members. T F

| Practitioner | Scoring Details | My Score |
|---|---|---|
| 1. **Fitness Yogi** | 3 pts. per "True" answer for 2, 5, 8, 13, 15 (*12 pts. or more signifies a fitness orientation)* | |
| 2. **Health-and-Healing Yogi** | 3 pts. per "True" answer for 4, 7, 11, 14, 19 (*12 pts. or more signifies a health-and-healing orientation)* | |
| 3. **Spiritual Yogi** | 3 pts. per "True" answer for 3, 6, 10, 12, 16 (*12 pts. or more signifies a spiritual orientation)* | |
| | ***Or maybe you're a . . .*** | |
| 4. **Yogi Mutt** | *(Scores of 12 or more for at least two of the three types)* | |
| 5. **Middle of the Roady Yogi** | *(Scores of less than 12 for each of the three types)* | |

# Appendix B

# Questions for Reflection: A Reader's Guide

## Introduction

How was I introduced to yoga? What influenced me to try it? What do I like about it?

## Chapter 1

What motivates me to practice yoga? What motivates others I know? How are the classes I take geared to my approach to yoga? Do they address more than physical aspects? Did the self-test in appendix A define my place in the yoga subculture? How or how not?

## Chapter 2

How does the "business" of yoga in my area affect my practice? How seriously are focused attention and breath awareness, chanting and meditation, and psychological or philosophical teachings entertained at the places where I take classes?

## Chapter 3

Do I wish to broaden or deepen my approach to Yoga? If I visit a yoga conference, retreat center, or new studio, what makes me feel at home? What, if anything, makes me feel unsettled? What are my expectations when choosing to visit?

## Chapter 4

Does yoga spirituality resonate with me? Why or why not? If interested, where could I practice it as part of a community? Have I checked out the authenticity of the practices provided there? Can I practice with my motivation in mind but without concern for reaching a particular outcome?

## Chapter 5

In what ways is yoga more a source of entertainment than a process for examining myself more deeply? How could I deepen my understanding of practices like devotional chanting? Can I participate in kirtan with a proper intention in mind?

## Chapter 6

Do my health professionals acknowledge the role of yoga in healing and preventive care? Are they aware that there is something more to yoga than feeling better or acting as a healing modality? How important is it to me that they acknowledge or respect the deeper side of yoga?

## Chapter 7

Does my practice of Yoga make any difference in how I conduct my daily life? How can I learn more about Yoga's role in my happiness? Does yoga act in concert with religious beliefs I hold?

## Chapter 8

How committed am I to "feel-good physicality" as the only outcome of doing yoga? What books or other resources can provide me with deeper understandings of what Yoga offers?

## Chapter 9

When a critical life change causes an upheaval in my life, how might I take it as an opportunity for self-exploration? Might I practice Yoga more regularly to embrace that opportunity?

## Chapter 10

To what degree is my practice and commitment to yoga characterized by the word *love*? Do I occasionally reflect on Yoga's role in my life and my evolving relationship to its practice?

## Chapter 11

To what extent is the love I express to others free of expecting something in return? How are my feelings of love connected to dependency and attachment rather than openness and nondiscrimination? Do I feel empathy and support from my teacher? Should I expect to?

## Chapter 12

What expectations do I bring to the yoga classes I take or teach? What do I expect from my teacher? Do I consciously focus on sensations and "own" any feelings that arise in class? How do I acknowledge expectations, feelings, and sensations during Yoga practice? How can I apply the yamas or niyamas to what happens in my asana class?

## Chapter 13

In simple ways, how can I show selfless service toward others—in and out of the yoga classes I take? How do I show appreciation for kindness I receive? Can I give without concern for the benefits that I accrue by giving? How can I surrender outcomes of my practice and offer their benefit to others?

## Chapter 14

Am I committed to work with my mind as I practice asanas? Where I do place my attention? Do I work with my breath? How might I practice these aspects of Yoga out in the world?

## Chapter 15

In what ways do I feel a sense of personal or spiritual progress through Yoga? Does my teacher "prepare the ground" for my transformation? If not, where can I find a teacher who can?

## Chapter 16

How does my practice embody the notion of tapas? When I ramp up my yoga practice, am I motivated more by physical goals than self-exploration? How are these motivations related?

## Chapter 17

Who in my life is having a difficult time right now? How can I make myself available to them? Might a yoga retreat help me work on the personal issues of greatest importance to me? How can I apply the meanings inherent in the yamas and niyamas to my life experience so they become a natural manifestation of both my life and my practice?

## Chapter 18

Do I have a pattern of mindlessly chasing my desires that only creates trouble for me? What would be a healthier way to acknowledge, accept, and integrate them? How can Yoga practice help me understand them more deeply?

## Chapter 19

How can self-study become a larger and more regular part of my own life? Once I identify a particular "poison," what are ways to apply "antidotes" that help loosen their hold on me?

## Chapter 20

Where does my sense of bliss—my life purpose—lie? How can I make it more central to my life? If I am living my bliss, how can I influence others to explore theirs?

## Chapter 21

What transformative stories that I read or hear about attract me? What myth, fairy tale, or film best embodies the heroic developments in my own life? What do I need to begin my own transformation right now—to become happier, healthier, freer, and of greater service to others?

## Chapter 22

How might I more regularly contemplate my ever-changing life, even when I am feeling stuck? What would make me better prepared for death—mine or that of someone I care about? How is that preparation the same as living my life more fully?

## Conclusion

How can I commit to practice Yoga more deeply? How can I promote or contribute to a more spirit-based Yoga in my community—through an investment of time, energy, or money?

APPENDIX C

# North American Centers for Practice and Study

While many yoga centers provide deeper teachings associated with Yoga, the following retreat centers offer residential and nonresidential programs for pursuing yoga practice as a holistic lifestyle. The types of accommodations and prices vary, as do the nature and length of programs.

**Arkansas**

| | |
|---|---|
| Fayetteville | *Wattle Hollow Retreat Center*<br>http://www.wattlehollow.com |

**California**

| | |
|---|---|
| Big Sur | *Esalen Institute*<br>http://www.esalen.org |
| Carlsbad | *Chopra Center for Wellbeing*<br>http://www.chopra.com |
| Costa Mesa | *Yoga Center Mountain Retreat*<br>http://www.yogacenter.org |
| Davis | *The Bo Tree: Yoga for Everyone*<br>http://www.thebotree.com |
| Grass Valley | *Sivananda Ashram Yoga Farm*<br>http://www.yogafarm.org |
| Los Angeles | *Atma Yoga Ashram*<br>http://yogamandir.com |
| Nevada City | *The Expanding Light: Ananda Yoga and Meditation Retreat Center*<br>http://www.expandinglight.org |

Santa Barbara — *White Lotus Foundation*
http://www.whitelotus.org

Santa Rosa — *Ananda Seva Mission*
http://www.anandaseva.org

Tomales — *Blue Mountain Center of Meditation*
http://www.easwaran.org

Watsonville — *Mt. Madonna Center*
http://www.mountmadonna.org

**Colorado**

Boulder — *Eldorado Mountain Yoga Ashram*
http://www.eldoradoyoga.org

Red Feather Lakes — *Shambhala Mountain Center*
http://www.shambhalamountain.org

Rollinsville — *Shoshoni Yoga Retreat*
http://www.shoshoni.org

**Florida**

Salt Springs — *Amrit Yoga Institute*
http://amrityoga.org

**Georgia**

Lakemont — *Center for Spiritual Awareness*
http://www.csa-davis.org

**Hawaii**

Hilo — *Kalani Oceanside Retreat*
http://www.kalani.com

Kealakekua — *Big Island Yoga Center of Hawaii*
http://www.bigislandyoga.com

Pahoa — *Yoga Oasis*
http://www.yogaoasis.org

**Indiana**

Mauckport — *Orbis Farm*
http://www.orbisfarm.com

**Massachusetts**

Lenox — *Kripalu Center for Yoga and Health*
http://www.kripalu.org

**Michigan**

| | |
|---|---|
| Vanderbilt | *Golden Lotus & Song of the Morning Center*<br>http://www.goldenlotus.org |

**Montana**

| | |
|---|---|
| Helena | *Feathered Pipe Ranch*<br>http://www.featheredpipe.com |

**New Hampshire**

| | |
|---|---|
| Hampton | *Institute for Personal Development*<br>*Kriya Yoga Ashram*<br>http://www.ipdtransform.com |

**New York**

| | |
|---|---|
| Monroe | *Ananda Ashram*<br>http://anandaashram.org |
| New York | *Dharma Mittra Yoga Center*<br>http://www.dharmayogacenter.com |
| Rhinebeck | *Omega Institute*<br>http://www.eomega.org |
| South Fallsburg | *Siddha Yoga/Shree Muktananda Ashram*<br>http://siddhayoga.org |
| Woodbourne | *Sivananda Ashram Yoga Ranch*<br>http://www.sivananda.org/ranch |

**North Carolina**

| | |
|---|---|
| Columbus | *DeerHaven Hills Farm & Yoga Eco-Center*<br>http://www.dhhf.org |

**Pennsylvania**

| | |
|---|---|
| Honesdale | *Himalayan Institute*<br>http://www.himalayaninstitute.org |
| West Sunbury | *Datta Yoga Retreat Center*<br>http://www.dycusa.org |

**Rhode Island**

| | |
|---|---|
| Hopkinton | *Ananda Retreat Center*<br>http://www.anandaeast.org |

**Tennessee**

| | |
|---|---|
| Hohenwald | *Gray Bear Holistic Retreat Center*<br>http://www.graybear.org |

### Texas

| | |
|---|---|
| Austin | *AYA Yoga and Meditation Center / Advaita Yoga Ashrama*<br>http://yoga108.org/pages/show/25 |
| | *Barsana Dham Yoga Ashram and Retreat Center*<br>http://www.barsanadham.org |

### Utah

| | |
|---|---|
| Brian Head | *Inner Harmony Yoga Retreat*<br>http://www.innerharmonyyoga.com |

### Virginia

| | |
|---|---|
| Buckingham | *Yogaville Satchidananda Ashram*<br>http://www.yogaville.org |

### Washington

| | |
|---|---|
| Greenbank | *The Yoga Lodge on Whidbey Island*<br>http://www.yogalodge.com |
| Vaughn | *Amrita Meditation Retreat Center*<br>http://ajayan.com |

## CANADA

### British Columbia

| | |
|---|---|
| Cortes Bay | *Hollyhock*<br>http://www.hollyhock.bc.ca |
| Kootenay Bay | *Yasodhara Ashram Yoga Retreat and Study Center*<br>http://www.yasodhara.org |
| Salmon Arm | *Ishana Retreat and Yoga Center*<br>http://www.ishana.org |
| Salt Spring Island | *Salt Spring Centre of Yoga*<br>*Ganges Yoga Studio*<br>http://www.saltspringcentre.com/enter.htm |

### Quebec

| | |
|---|---|
| St-Etienne-De-Bolton | *Babaji's Kriya Yoga Ashram*<br>http://www.babaji.ca |
| Val-Morin | *Sivananda Ashram Yoga Camp–Quebec*<br>http.www.sivananda.org |

# NOTES

## Preface

1. For books on the practice of Yoga as a spiritual discipline, see the bibliography.

2. Stephen Cope, *Will Yoga and Meditation Really Change My Life?* (North Adams, MA: Storey Publishing, 2003). This engaging work highlights twenty-five prominent yoga and meditation teachers, only two of whom reside in the vast area between the Rockies and the Appalachians. In 2003, the International Association of Yoga Therapists noted on the other hand that fully 50 percent of yoga practitioners in America live between the Northeastern and West Coast states. See www.namasta.com.

## Introduction

1. *Yoga Journal*'s poll by Harris Interactive noted that Americans spend $5.7 billion on yoga classes, products, and services and that 15.8 million adults practiced yoga by 2008, declining slightly since 2005. Half are newcomers, practicing for two years or less. See "Yoga Journal Releases 2008 'Yoga in America Market Study,'" www.yogajournal.com, February 26, 2008.

2. Mediamark Research notes that the number of "frequent practitioners" (taking at least two classes a week) more than doubled from 1.3 million in 2001 to about 3 million in 2006. See Rachel Konrad, "Yoga Stretches into the Public Schools," Associated Press release, January 28, 2007.

3. Pandit Rajmani Tigunait, September 25, 2000, interview with Rod Stryker, www.pureyoga.com.

4. See John Capouya, "Real Men Do Yoga," *Newsweek*, June 16, 2003.

5. See Dr. Timothy McCall, *Yoga as Medicine: The Yogic Prescription for Health and Healing* (New York: Bantam, 2007), 493, where he argues that "the growing interest in yoga and its applications to health has come from the general public, not the medical profession—in part because people weren't getting the answers and the help they needed from their doctors or other health care providers."

6. For a list of books on yoga from a fitness or health perspective, see the bibliography.

7. For two fine descriptions of the story of Ramakrishna and Vivekananda, see Stephen Cross, *Way of Hinduism* (London: Thorsons, 2002) and Elisabeth De Michelis, *A History of Modern Yoga* (London: Continuum, 2004). The latter provides a detailed description of forms of modern yoga in the United Kingdom that mirror developments in America. For an entertaining journalistic history of American yoga, see Robert Love, "Fear of Yoga," *Columbia Journalism Review*, November/December 2006. Linda Sparrowe covers yoga developments in California in *Yoga, A Yoga Journal Book* (Fairfield, CT: Levin, Hugh Lauter Associates, 2004).

8. Krishnamacharya's quotation appears in the preface to Mark Forstater and Jo Manuel, *Yoga Masters* (New York: Penguin Putnam, 2002).

## Chapter 1: Yoga Class, Culture Clash

1. De Michelis, *A History of Modern Yoga*, 252 (see introduction, n. 7).

2. Georg Feuerstein, *The Shambhala Guide to Yoga* (Boston: Shambhala, 1996), 26.

3. Srivatsa Ramaswami and David Hurwitz, *Yoga Beneath the Surface* (New York: Marlowe and Company, 2006), 204–5.

4. De Michelis, *A History of Modern Yoga*, 251.

5. Feuerstein, *The Shambhala Guide to Yoga*, 69.

6. Ramaswami and Hurwitz, *Yoga Beneath the Surface*, 205.

7. Ibid., 206.

8. Marina Budhos, "Culture Shock," *Yoga Journal*, June 2002, 166.

9. Clare Duffy, event transcript, "Spirit Wars: American Religion in Progressive Politics," Key West, Florida, December 6, 2005. See http://pewforum.org/events.

## Chapter 2: An American Revolution

*Epigraph.* Geeta Iyengar, in Budhos, "Culture Shock," 167 (see chap. 1, n. 8).

1. For an excellent history of yoga, see Linda Sparrowe, *Yoga, A Yoga Journal Book* (see introduction, n. 7).

2. Fernando Pages Ruiz explores Krishnamacharya's influence on American yoga in "Krishnamacharya's Legacy," *Yoga Journal*, June 2001.

3. Ann Pizer, *Your Guide to Yoga*, http://yoga.about.com/poweryoga/a/power.htm, November 30, 2005.

4. In a 2006 national survey by the Pew Research Center, 55 percent of eighteen-to-thirty-nine-year-olds identified the most important goal for their age group as getting rich, while 11 percent said it was to become more spiritual. Being famous came in second (30 percent).

5. Carina Chocano, "The Allure of Illusion," *Los Angeles Times*, May 21, 2006.

6. Ramaswami and Hurwitz, *Yoga Beneath the Surface*, 205 (see chap. 1, n. 3).

7. See David Eisenberg et al., "Unconventional Medicine in the United States: Prevalence, Costs and Patterns of Use," *New England Journal of Medicine*, 328 (1993): 246–52 and "Trends in Alternative Medicine Use in the United States, 1990–1997," *Journal of the American Medical Association* (*JAMA*) 280 (1998): 1569–75.

8. Anne Cushman, "Has the Commercialization of Spiritual Life Gone Too Far?" www.yogajournal.com, December 19, 2005.

9. Tara Guber's "Yoga Ed" program and quotes from Christian writers are described in Rachel Konrad, "Yoga Stretches into the Public Schools," Associated Press release, January 28, 2007.

10. "Stretching for Jesus" in *Time*, August 29, 2005, led to a response by Swaminathan Venkataraman and Mihir Meghani on behalf of the Hindu American Foundation.

11. See Richard Corliss, "The Power of Yoga," *Time*, April 15, 2001, and Josh Ulick, "Yoga and Massage: If It's Physical, It's Therapy," *Newsweek*, December 2, 2002.

12. "Has Hollywood's Yoga Obsession Gone Too Far?" *US Weekly*, March 31, 2003, appeared at Baron Baptiste's Power Yoga Institute Web site: www.baron baptiste.com.

13. "Yoga's Bad Boy: Bikram Choudhury," www.yogajournal.com, December 19, 2005. Recent articles question the positive health effects of Bikram yoga; see "When Does Flexible Become Harmful? 'Hot' Yoga Draws Fire," *New York Times*, March 30, 2004.

14. The NAMASTA estimate was cited at www.namasta.com.

15. Rod Stryker with Pandit Rajmani Tigunait, www.pureyoga.com, September 25, 2000.

16. *Yoga Journal's* magazine and Web site advertise its travel cruises. Also see Debra Klein on upscale vacations in "Inner Peace, Good Eats!" *Newsweek*, March 18, 2002, and Nirmala Nataraj on Cyndi Lee's experiences in "The Travels of a Yogi," *Yogi Times*, May 2005.

17. See www.americansportsdata.com, April 4, 2003.

18. See "Hollywood Stars Fall in Love with Yoga during Pregnancy," Health, Beauty and Fitness Center Web site, www.luvcube.com, July 15, 2005.

19. Georg Feuerstein, *The Deeper Dimension of Yoga: Theory and Practice* (Boston: Shambhala, 2003), 239.

20. J. Brown, "The Making of a Yoga Therapy Center, Part 1," *Yoga Therapy in Practice,* March 2008.

21. See Steven Waldman and Valerie Reiss, "Beliefwatch: Lohasians," *Newsweek*, June 5, 2006 and Ariana Speyer, "Riding the Metrospiritual Wave," www.beliefnet.com/story/177.

22. John Abbott, "Yoga Journal Releases 'Yoga in America' Market Study," www.yogajournal.com, February 7, 2005.

23. Deborah Willoughby, "Editor's Letter," *Yoga + Joyful Living*, July–August 2006, 6.

24. An online yoga survey "Yoga Now," sponsored by the Yoga Site, Inc. in the late 1990s, found that the typical practitioner was "a woman in her mid-thirties who does yoga three to five times a week, has been practicing for less than two years, and believes in reincarnation." Most practice it as a mental and/or fitness regimen. Given recent demographic trends toward young practitioners, the average practitioner age may have declined slightly from that of thirty-four reported by Yoga Site, Inc.

25. While alternative publications often cover yoga, three examples of mainstream coverage of yoga's hybridization are the fusion of yoga with rafting, laughter, surfing, and snowboarding. See Laura Bly, "Rafting that Stretches the Boundaries," *USA Today,* August 15, 2003; Jennifer Saranow, "Health: Latest Hybrid Yoga Encourages Giggling toward a Higher Plane," *Wall Street Journal,* October 13, 2004; and Jane Margolies, "Everybody Calm? Let's Surf!" *New York Times,* July 24, 2005.

    Americanization affects Hinduism as well, as reflected in pop culture's twisted meanings associated with concepts like "karma" or "dharma." See "Hindu Lite: Pop Culture Plays Fast and Loose with an Ancient Faith," *USA Today*, February 16, 2006.

26. Srivatsa Ramaswami, "My Studies With Sri Krishnamacharya," *Namarupa*, Spring 2007, 21.

27. Cushman, "Has the Commercialization of Spiritual Life . . ." (see n. 8).

## CHAPTER 3: FILLING THE BIG TENT

1. Organizers of the Yoga in Toronto Conference and Show cite this data from

PMB, Harris Interactive Service Bureau, and *Yoga Journal* Demographic Information. See www.yogaintoronto.com.

2. See Stephen Cope, *Yoga and the Search for the True Self* (New York: Bantam, 1999) for an excellent description of the spiritual origins and organizational transformation of Kripalu Center for Yoga and Health. His discussion of "transformational space" on pp. 26–32 is especially pertinent.

## Chapter 4: Making It on Broadway

1. See Waldman and Reiss, "Beliefwatch: Lohasians," *Newsweek* (chap. 2, n. 21).
2. Ariana Speyer, "Riding the Metrospiritual Wave," www.beliefnet.com, 3.
3. Lama Yeshe, *Introduction to Tantra: A Vision of Totality* (Boston: Wisdom Publications, 1987), 144.

## Chapter 5: Temple and Club

1. Krist Novoselic, "Interview with Krishna Das," www.samadhi-yoga.com, September 15, 2005, 2.
2. See Atma Jo Ann Levitt, comp. and ed., *Pilgrim of Love: The Life and Teachings of Swami Kripalu* (Rhinebeck, NY: Monkfish, 2004), 179.
3. Novoselic, "Interview with Krishna Das," 4.
4. Levitt, *Pilgrim of Love,* 179.
5. Novoselic, "Interview with Krishna Das," 2.

## Chapter 6: The Crossroads

1. On the annual production of new allopathic physicians, see Mryle Croasdale, "Physician Work Force Estimates Far Apart," June 20, 2005, at *amednews.com,* a newspaper for U.S. physicians.
2. Journals such as *Alternative Therapies in Health and Science* were established in the mid-1990s in response to growing professional and public interest. They have focused on nonallopathic therapies ranging from indigenous healing to chiropractic modalities. Later in the decade, the *Journal of the American Medical Association* began to run articles examining complementary and alternative care in medical schools while exploring yoga's efficacy as a treatment modality for specific conditions. In *JAMA,* see Garfinkel et al., "Yoga-Based Intervention for Carpal Tunnel Syndrome: A Randomized Trial," 280 (1998): 1601–03; Daniell et al., "Yoga for Carpal Tunnel Syndrome," 281 (1999): 2087–89.

3. Meditation, encompassing part of Classical Yoga's eight limbs of practice, has also been subjected to empirical science's research methodology with growing interest in its positive effect on well-being. See coverage of research studies conducted at the University of Wisconsin in Katherine Combes, "Study Shows Positive Impact of Meditation on Brain, Anti-Bodies," *The Epoch Times*, May 31, 2004.
4. Ramaswami and Hurwitz, *Yoga Beneath the Surface*, 205–6 (see chap. 1, n. 3).
5. Excellent examples of the role of yoga professionals in merging scientific rigor with yoga spirituality are found in publications of the International Association of Yoga Therapists, including its *International Journal of Yoga Therapy* and its newsletter, *Yoga Therapy in Practice*. Such work often grounds yoga's seemingly esoteric concepts in explorations of their relationship to concrete, psychophysical conditions.
6. Chase Bossart, "Yoga Bodies, Yoga Minds: How Indian Anatomies Form the Foundation of Yoga for Healing," *International Journal of Yoga Therapy* 17 (2007): 27.
7. Joseph Le Page, "The Future of Yoga Therapy," *Yoga Therapy in Practice* 3, no. 1 (March 2007): 21.
8. Feuerstein, *The Deeper Dimension of Yoga*, 28 (see chap. 2, n. 19).

## Chapter 7: Indian Interlude

1. Georg Feuerstein receives credit for capitalizing the word *Yoga* to highlight it as a spiritual path in Donna Farhi, *Bringing Yoga to Life* (San Francisco: HarperCollins, 2004).

## Chapter 8: Twisted

1. The film *What the Bleep Do We Know!?* (Twentieth Century Fox, 2004) drew on the insights of quantum physics and New Age spirituality to propose that there is no solid reality, since reality is intimately affected by our changing perceptions and intentions. The sixty-page online study guide on these issues, sponsored by the Institute of Noetic Sciences and Captured Light Industries, serves as a springboard for exploring assumptions common to both physics and Yoga.
2. H. David Coulter's *Anatomy of Hatha Yoga* (Honesdale, PA: Body and Breath Inc, 2001) provides in-depth anatomical aspects of Hatha yoga postures and is an excellent resource for teachers and students alike. This chapter relies on his informative discussion of twisting postures, 383–486.

# Notes

## Chapter 9: Promise and Fruition

*Epigraph*: Rig Veda 1.164.37.

1. Abraham Maslow refers to peak experiences throughout his work. See especially *Religions, Values, and Peak-Experiences* (New York: Viking, 1964).
2. Georg Feuerstein, *Tantra: The Path of Ecstasy* (Boston: Shambhala, 2003), 253.
3. Stephen Cope, *The Wisdom of Yoga* (New York: Bantam, 2006), 126.

## Chapter 10: An Unconditional Opening

*Epigraph:* Swami Sai Premananda, *Principles of Higher Living: The Western Experience upon the Shores of Eastern Wisdom* (Mississauga, ON: Moksha Publishing, 2006), 92.

1. For a behavioral science investigation of styles of loving, see Marcia Lasswell and Thomas Lasswell, *Marriage and the Family* (New York: Wadsworth, 1991).
2. Feuerstein, *The Deeper Dimension of Yoga*, 277 (see chap. 2, n. 19).
3. B. K. S. Iyengar, *Yoga: The Path to Holistic Health* (London: Dorling Kindersley, 2001), 155.
4. The oft-noted quotation by Albert Camus fully reads, "Man must live and create. Live to the point of tears" (source unknown).
5. The idea of "spiritual warriorship" occurs in many traditions, most recently in the Shambhala tradition of Tibetan Buddhism as articulated by the late Chögyam Trungpa Rinpoche.

## Chapter 12: Body, Mind, and Teacher

*Epigraph:* Donna Farhi, *Teaching Yoga* (Berkeley: Rodmell Press, 2006), 15.

1. The psychotherapeutic principles informing this chapter are generic assumptions many therapists make in working with couples on communication issues. They are also evident in the award-winning Couple Communication Program trademarked by Interpersonal Communication Programs, Inc. of Evergreen, Colorado. Its work is among the most researched in the area of marriage education. See S. F. Jakubowski, et al., "A review of empirically supported marital enrichment programs," *Family Relations* 53 (2004): 528–536.
2. Rod Stryker in discussion with Pandit Rajmani Tigunait (see chap. 2, n. 15).

## CHAPTER 13: ZERO GRAVITY

*Epigraph:* Source unknown according to the *Los Angeles Times*, July 30, 1989.

1. The American Obesity Association (AOA) categorizes 64.5 percent of all adult Americans as overweight or obese. Sixty-two percent of women aged twenty to seventy-four are overweight; 34 percent are obese (with a Body Mass Index of 30 or more). The National Center for Health Statistics notes that, from the early 1960s to the year 2000, obesity among women aged thirty-five to forty-four jumped from 15 to 34 percent; aged forty-five to fifty-four, from 20 to 38 percent; and aged fifty-five to sixty-four, from 24 to 43 percent. See AOA's Web site, www.obesity.org.

2. Nicholas Christakis of the Harvard Medical School and James Fowler of the University of California at San Diego affirmed the role of Americans' social networks in influencing the spread of obesity through the development of norms that consider it acceptable. See the *New England Journal of Medicine* 357, no. 4 (2007): 370–79.

## CHAPTER 14: THE GENTLE REBELLION

*Epigraph:* Maitri Upanishad 6:22:26.

1. Translations of the sutras of Patanjali vary from writer to writer. This chapter borrows from Barbara Stoler Miller, *Yoga: Discipline of Freedom: The Yoga Sutra Attributed to Patanjali* (New York: Bantam, 1998).

2. The quote is by Katsuaki Watanabe, President of Toyota, and concerns innovation in international business. See *Expanding the Innovation Horizon: The Global CEO Study 2006* (New York: IBM Corporation, 2006), 32.

3. Paramahansa Yogananda, *Inner Reflections: Selections from the Writings of Paramahansa Yogananda* (Los Angeles: Self-Realization Fellowship, 2007), unpaginated calendar.

4. Lois Nesbitt, "An Insomniac Awakes," in Valerie Jeremijenko, *How to Live Our Yoga* (Boston: Beacon Press, 2001), 104.

5. Farhi, *Bringing Yoga to Life*, 130–31 (see chap. 7, n. 1).

6. There are slight differences in how authors describe and interpret the sheaths. I draw upon Feuerstein, *The Shambhala Guide to Yoga,* 70 (see chap. 1, n. 2).

7. Farhi, *Bringing Yoga to Life,* 89.

8. Ibid.

## Chapter 15: Primordial Nature

*Epigraph:* Ramaswami and Hurwitz, *Yoga Beneath the Surface*, 156 (see chap. 1, n. 3).

1. The profile of yoga practitioners as young, professional, arts and fitness oriented, female, and liberal was consistent in two unpublished studies at the beginning of the yoga boom in the United States: the MDI Lifestyle Survey (Wisconsin, 1996) and the national Yoga Site Inc. survey (1998).
2. See Paul Ray and Sherry Anderson, *Cultural Creatives: How 50 Million People Are Changing the World* (New York: Harmony, 2000). It is likely that their concept includes many yoga practitioners, especially those committed to holistic health.
3. Lilian Silburn, *Kundalini: The Energy of the Depths* (Albany: State University of New York Press, 1988), xiv. For techniques in the guru's piercing of the student's energy centers, see 87–101.
4. Daniel Odier, *Desire: The Tantric Path to Awakening* (Rochester, VT: Inner Traditions, 2001), 48.
5. Rammurti Mishra, *Fundamentals of Yoga* (New York: Three Rivers, 1987), 1.
6. At first, I was reluctant to share my own experience with Yoga in this book. Eastern traditions warn followers about the subtle undermining influence of ego on one's personal progress, especially concerning experiences meant only for one's spiritual guide. Yet I myself am engaged more deeply by personal accounts of individual yogis than by abstract descriptions. So, rightly or wrongly, I include a few of my own—not as some measure of personal accomplishment—but as evidence that the practice of American Yoga as a lifestyle can lead us to affirm the wisdom of Yoga's ancient teachings. They are open to anyone dedicated to the path, and the experiences described are indeed possible for anyone to attain.
7. Feuerstein, *The Shambhala Guide to Yoga,* 49 (see chap. 1, n. 2).
8. Yeshe, *Introduction to Tantra*, 139 (see chap. 4, n. 3).
9. Silburn, *Kundalini,* 28.
10. Swami Muktananada in Ajit Mookerjee, *Kundalini: The Arousal of the Inner Energy* (Rochester, VT: Destiny, 1986), 73.
11. Silburn, *Kundalini*, 26.
12. Ibid.
13. Yogananda, *Inner Reflections* (see chap. 14, n. 3).
14. Feuerstein, *The Deeper Dimension of Yoga*, 126 (see chap. 2, n. 19).

## CHAPTER 17: EMILY'S HEART

1. For a guide to the wide range of yoga vacations, see Jenne Ricci, *Yoga Escapes* (Berkeley: Celestial Arts, 2003).

2. Some American sexual-assault treatment facilities apply Kübler-Ross's stages of grief—denial, anger, depression, bargaining, and acceptance—to the experience of rape survivors. The award-winning DVD/cassette program *Surviving Rape: A Journey through Grief* (Boston: Fanlight Productions, 1992) is a powerful resource. In it, as the program materials state, five rape survivors "recall their experiences of rape and subsequent grief. Although each woman's road to recovery was different, they all shared feelings of shame, self-hatred, and guilt before finally reaching acceptance and self-love. These survivors stress the importance of talking about their trauma and seeking help from a support group to begin the healing process."

3. Elisabeth Kübler-Ross and David Kessler, *On Grief and Grieving* (New York: Scribner, 2005), 81–82.

4. Laureen Smith, "Yoga and the Healing Journey: From Sexual Abuse to Wholeness," *Yoga Studies: A Newsletter of the International Association of Yoga Therapists* 13 (January–April 2003): 5.

5. Pema Chödrön, *The Places that Scare You: A Guide to Fearlessness in Difficult Times* (Boston: Shambhala, 2001), 82.

6. Ibid.

## CHAPTER 18: INDRA'S NET

*Epigraph:* Yogananda, *Inner Reflections* (see chap. 14, n. 3).

1. Marie-Louise Von Franz, *On Divination and Synchronicity: The Psychology of Meaningful Chance* (Toronto: Inner City, 1980), 39–40.

2. Ibid., 84.

3. Ibid., 102.

4. Mark Epstein, *Open to Desire: Embracing a Lust for Life* (New York: Penguin, 2005), 41.

5. Ibid., 111.

6. For Joseph Campbell's discussion of love, see his *The Power of Myth* with Bill Moyers, Betty Sue Flowers, ed. (New York: Doubleday, 1988), 184–205.

## Chapter 19: Poison and Antidote

1. The Associated Press announced these statistics on December 15, 2004, according to the trade publication *Pollstar*.
2. Interview with Barry Egan, *Sunday Independent*, January 2004, www.sting.com.
3. In *The Deeper Dimension of Yoga*, chapter 45 (see chap. 2, n. 19), Feuerstein points out that the "three poisons" appear in both Hindu and Buddhist Yoga, with attachment replacing greed in some Buddhist teachings.
4. Sting, *Broken Music* (New York: Random House, 2003), 324.
5. Interview with Neil McCormick, *The Daily Telegraph*, September 2003, www.sting.com.
6. Sting discussed his meditative labyrinth on David Dye's World Café, National Public Radio, November 24, 2006.
7. Stephen Dalton, "Sting has been stung by the yoga bug—and his life will never be the same," *Yoga Journal*, December 1995, www.sting.com.

## Chapter 20: Water So Pure and Clear

*Epigraph:* Katha Upanishad, 2:1:10.

1. Miller, *Yoga: Discipline of Freedom*, 60 (see chap. 14, n. 1).
2. Ibid., 67.
3. Campbell with Moyers, *The Power of Myth*, 120 (see chap. 18, n. 6).
4. Ibid., 148–49.
5. Ravi Ravindra, *The Spiritual Roots of Yoga* (Sandpoint, ID: Morning Light Press, 2006), 6.
6. Campbell with Moyers, *The Power of Myth*, 118–19.

## Chapter 21: Elephant-Headed

1. Stories of Ganesha appear throughout India and in many ancient scriptural works as well as modern studies of myth. One splendid resource is the chapter "The Divine Family of Shiva" in Namita Gokhale, *The Book of Shiva* (New Delhi: Penguin, 2001).
2. Royina Grewal, *The Book of Ganesha* (New Delhi: Penguin, 2001), 12.

## CHAPTER 22: LAST BREATH

*Epigraph:* from the weekly e-mail message sent by Babaji's Kriya Yoga Ashram, St. Etienne de Bolton, Quebec, November 12, 2004.

1. Ram Dass, *Still Here: Embracing Aging, Changing, and Dying* (New York: Riverhead Books, 2000), 181–82.
2. Ibid., 161.
3. Ibid., 170.
4. For an excellent description of Tantric practices for death and the dying, see Sogyal Rinpoche, *The Tibetan Book of Living and Dying* (New York: HarperCollins, 1992).

## CONCLUSION

1. Swami Sivananda's extensive interpretations of dream symbols appear at www.experiencefestival.com.
2. Swami Vishnu Tirtha, *Devatma Shakti: Divine Power* (Varanasi: Government Sanskrit College, 1962), 147.
3. See Joseph Campbell, *Pathways to Bliss: Mythology and Personal Transformation* (Novato, CA: New World Library, 2004), 124–26.
4. Ramaswami and Hurwitz, *Yoga Beneath the Surface*, 156 (see chap. 1, n. 3).

# BIBLIOGRAPHY

## Yoga as a Spiritual Discipline

Since the 1960s, an accumulated body of published work in English has addressed yoga spirituality and the depth and breadth of practice as a spiritual discipline. These often range from scholarly analyses to spiritual treatises. Since this exploration of the world of yoga is neither, I provide below only a few of the many resources written by authoritative authors, teachers, and scholars.

Chetanananda, Swami. *The Breath of God.* Cambridge: Rudra Press, 1990.

Cope, Stephen. *The Wisdom of Yoga: A Seeker's Guide to Extraordinary Living.* New York: Bantam, 2006.

Desikachar, T .K. V. *The Heart of Yoga: Developing a Personal Practice.* Rochester, VT: Integral Yoga Publications, 1999.

Farhi, Donna. *Bringing Yoga to Life: The Everyday Practice of Enlightened Living.* San Francisco: Harper, 2003.

Feuerstein, Georg. *The Deeper Dimension of Yoga: Theory and Practice.* Boston: Shambhala, 2003.

Gilbert, Elizabeth. *Eat, Pray, Love.* New York: Bantam, 2006.

Iyengar, B. K. S. *Light on Life: The Yoga Journey to Wholeness, Inner Peace and Ultimate Freedom.* New York: Rodale, 2005.

Iyengar, B. K. S. *Light on Yoga.* London: George Allen and Unwin, Ltd., 1966.

Muktananda, Swami and Swami Chidvilasananda. *Play of Consciousness: A Spiritual Autobiography.* San Francisco: Harper & Row, 1978.

Ramaswami, Srivatsa and David Hurwitz. *Yoga Beneath the Surface: An American Student and His Indian Teacher Discuss Yoga Philosophy and Practice.* New York: Marlowe, 2006.

Satchidananda, Sri Swami. *To Know Yourself.* Yogaville, VA: Integral Yoga Publications, 1999.

Yogananda, Paramahansa. *Autobiography of a Yogi.* Los Angeles: Self-Realization Fellowship, 1973.

## Yoga from a Fitness Perspective

More numerous than spiritually based works on yoga are those focused on Hatha practice from a fitness or health perspective. On June 1, 2008, a Google search for "yoga books" yielded over 1,210,000 entries. Most are likely to be "how-to" books. Here is a partial but representative list:

Austin, Miriam. *Cool Yoga Tricks.* New York: Ballantine, 2003.

———. *Yoga for Wimps.* New York: Sterling Publications, 1999.

Gallanis, Bess. *Yoga Chick: A Hip Guide to Everything Om.* New York: Time Warner, 2006.

Hittleman, Richard. *Yoga: A 28 Day Exercise Plan.* New York: Bantam Dell, 2004.

Lasater, Judith Hanson. *Yoga Abs: Moving from Your Core.* Berkeley: Rodmell Press, 2005.

Page, Diamond Dallas. *Yoga for Regular Guys: The Best Damn Workout on the Planet.* Philadelphia: Quirk Books, 2005.

Rentz, Kristen. *Yoga Nap: Restorative Poses for Deep Relaxation.* New York: Marlowe, 2005.

Rountree, Sage. *The Athlete's Guide to Yoga: An Integrated Approach to Strength, Flexibility and Focus.* Boulder, CO: Velo Press, 2008.

Twining, Glenda. *Yoga Fights Flab: A 30-Day Program to Tone, Trim, and Flatten Your Trouble Spots.* Gloucester, MA: Fair Winds Press, 2004.

Vilga, Edward. *Yoga in Bed: 20 Asanas to do in Pajamas.* Philadelphia: Running Press Books, 2005.

Yoga Journal's *Yoga Step-by-Step Home Practice System with Natasha Rizopoulos.* Boulder: Sounds True, 2004.

Zeer, Darrin. *Travel Yoga: Stretches for Planes, Trains, Automobiles and More!* San Francisco: Chronicle Books, 2005.

## YOGA FROM A HEALTH AND HEALING PERSPECTIVE

While "how-to" books often provide helpful, health-related information related to asana and pranayama practice, "health and healing" forms a specialized genre of yoga resources. The following are representative examples:

Blaine, Sandy. *Yoga for Healthy Knees: What You Need for Pain Prevention and Rehabilitation.* Berkeley: Rodmell Press, 2005.

Crotzer, Shoosh Lettick. *Yoga for Fibromyalgia.* Berkeley: Rodmell Press, 2008.

Epple, Anita and Pauline Carpenter. *Baby Massage and Yoga.* London: Hodder Headline, 2007.

Francina, Suza. *The New Yoga for Healthy Aging.* Deerfield, FL: Health Communications, Inc., 2007.

McCall, Timothy. *Yoga as Medicine: The Yogic Prescription for Health and Healing.* New York: Bantam, 2007.

Payne, Larry, and Richard Usatine. *Yoga Rx.* New York: Broadway Books, 2002.

# INDEX

# Index

# Index

# Index

# Quest Books

encourages open-minded inquiry into
world religions, philosophy, science, and the arts
in order to understand the wisdom of the ages,
respect the unity of all life, and help people explore
individual spiritual self-transformation.

Its publications are generously supported by
The Kern Foundation,
a trust committed to Theosophical education.

Quest Books is the imprint of
the Theosophical Publishing House,
a division of the Theosophical Society in America.
For information about programs, literature,
on-line study, membership benefits, and international centers,
see www.theosophical.org
or call 800-669-1571 or (outside the U.S.) 630-668-1571.

## Related Quest Titles

*Feng Shui for the Body*, by Daniel Santos

*The Meditative Path*, by John Cianciosi

*A Still Forest Pool*, by Jack Kornfield, with Paul Breiter

*Yoga for Your Spiritual Muscles*, by Rachel Schaeffer

*Zen Master Class*, by Stephen Hodge

To order books or a complete Quest catalog,
call 800-669-9425 or (outside the U.S.) 630-665-0130.